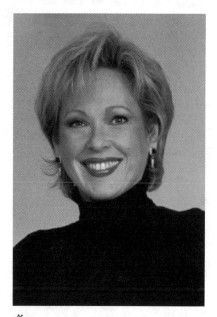

Janis Forbes Fite wanted to have her cake and eat it too. And she wanted Key lime pie, bearnaise sauce, pimiento cheese and other delicious foods.

But she knew that a high-fiber, low-fat diet was vital for her entire family, since both her mother and father had dealt with cancer. She knew the proper diet could reduce the risks for certain kinds of cancer as well as cardiovascular disease.

And she wanted to lose weight — permanently.

With the program of eating that she developed, she lost 20 pounds and she began to convert her friends.

Because of the program's effectiveness, word spread. People stayed with the program because their weight loss, like Fite's, was permanent — and because the food was good. Physicians began sending their patients to her.

Combining her credentials as a schoolteacher and a nurse, Fite developed Choices Unlimited classes and seminars. The program is also available in a two-tape video set. Her "students" wanted recipes as well as information.

The cookbook was written, as Fite says, "…that we all might eat cake!" Now her new volume II, she adds, "puts the icing on the cake."

Fite for Your Life II

more delicious high-fiber,
low-fat cookery
by
Janis Forbes Fite, R.N.

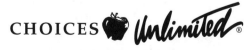

CHOICES Unlimited®

89 Stonehaven Drive
Jackson, Tennessee 38305

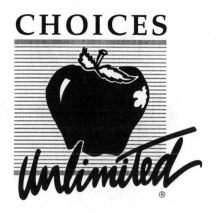

CHOICES
Unlimited ®

FIRST PRINTING — OCTOBER, 1996

ISBN # 0-9654322-1-1

Printed in the USA by

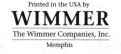

WIMMER
The Wimmer Companies, Inc.
Memphis

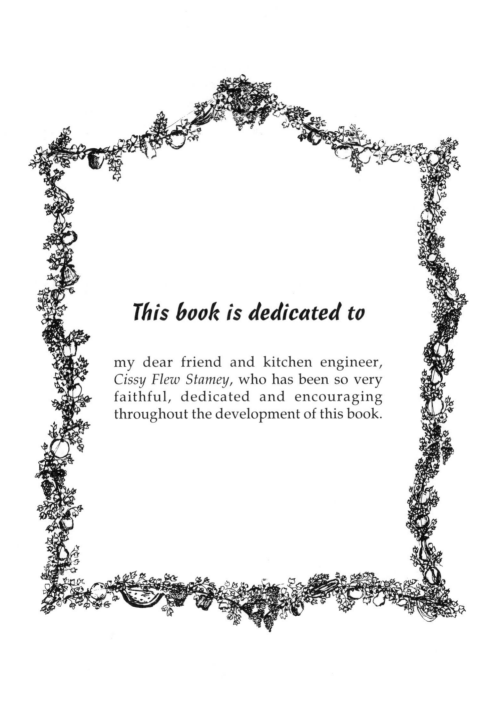

This book is dedicated to

my dear friend and kitchen engineer, *Cissy Flew Stamey*, who has been so very faithful, dedicated and encouraging throughout the development of this book.

The Choices Unlimited Program

COOKBOOK

The Choices Unlimited Program recognizes that we all need a practical approach to a *lifestyle* of healthy eating. This cookbook was written so that you can now enjoy your favorite foods without worry. For those of you who are following a therapeutic diet plan (i.e. American Diabetic Association's diet, etc.), we encourage you to adapt these recipes following your physician's guidelines.

VIDEO SET

This practical approach to high-fiber, low-fat eating is applied to dining-out, holidays, parties, and vacations in the **Fite For Your Life** video set. Also, understanding cholesterol and its relationship to food fats and fiber is made clear and easy in the video to assist you in achieving a healthy lifestyle.

PHILOSOPHY

Selecting a wide variety of high-fiber, low-fat foods from the seven food groups of the food pyramid, and drinking adequate amounts of water daily are keys to good nutrition.

Eating less fat reduces the amount of fat available for the body to store. Dietary fiber and regular aerobic exercise (as approved by your physician) contribute to releasing of fat already stored in the fat cells.

Choices Unlimited's version of the food pyramid is an updated version of the time-honored four basic food groups. The new approach consists of seven food groups:

1. Breads/Grains/Cereals - 6-11 servings daily
2. Vegetables - 3-5 servings daily
3. Fruits - 2-4 servings daily
4. Dairy - 2-4 servings daily
5. Meat/Meat Alternatives - 2-3 servings daily
6. Fats/Oils - limit to 1 fat gram per serving or per piece or per portion (excluding meat/meat alternatives which should not exceed 8 fat grams per serving)
7. Sugar (low-fat or fat-free sweets) in moderation, preferably eaten as desserts instead of between-meal snacks. This avoids a rapid rise in blood sugar which triggers insulin over-production, causing hormonal changes in women that can lead to more efficient fat storage.

Healthy eating is a choice. The Choices Unlimited Program makes that choice practical and enjoyable.

Happy and Healthy Eating!

Janis Fite

Table of Contents

Helpful Hints

When mixing fat-free cream cheese in a gelatin salad, it is important that you let the mixture of the gelatin and boiling water come to room temperature. In a separate bowl, add 2 tablespoons of gelatin mixture at a time to cream cheese and beat using a mixer until a smooth consistency is achieved after each addition. Then add remaining ingredients in recipe.

In selecting ground beef be sure to buy the new "lean" ground beefs.

If using homemade chicken or beef broth, skim fat by refrigerating until the fat is on top of broth, in solid form, for easy removal.

To sauté large amounts of vegetables such as onions, peppers, celery, etc., heat a non–stick skillet to medium–medium high heat. Afterward, spray skillet with Pam; add vegetables. Spray top of vegetables with Pam; cover. Stir periodically and keep covered. If skillet seems too "dry" spray again with Pam. If vegetables appear to start sweating, remove cover and continue cooking until crisp–tender.

When ground round or turkey, etc., is called for, crumble raw meat in a colander. Place colander in a microwave pie plate to "catch" fat. Place in microwave oven and cook 2–3 minutes. Remove and chop meat with a utensil. Return to microwave and repeat until done. Rinse under hot running water and drain well.
If a microwave is not available, cook in a skillet, then rinse under hot running water and drain well.

Use these recommended margarine products exactly as specified in each recipe for the best cooking and baking results:

> Fleischmann's Fat–free Squeezable Spread
> Ultra Promise Fat–free
> Ultra–Promise 70% Less Fat
> Butter Buds Liquid
> I Can't Believe It's Not Butter Spray

We do *not* recommend:

> I Can't Believe It's Not Butter Fat Free Tub Margarine
> Fleischmann's Fat Free Tub Margarine

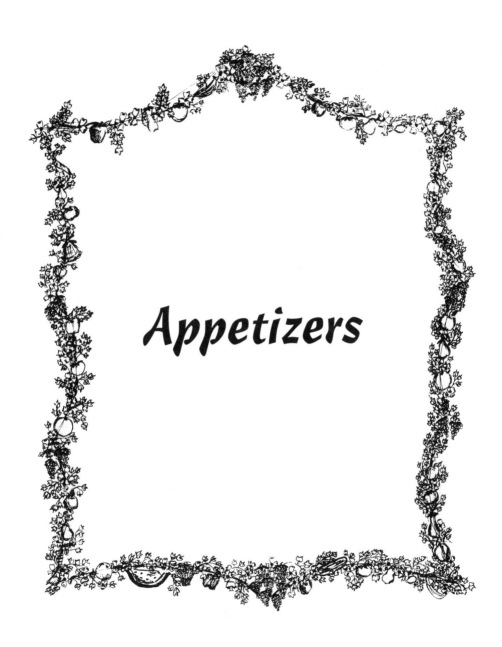

Appetizers

Assorted Finger Sandwiches

CHICKEN SALAD SANDWICHES:

Whole wheat bread, crusts removed

Chicken Salad (see page 142)

Spread trimmed bread with prepared chicken salad. Slice bread diagonally to make four triangles.

CRAB SALAD SANDWICHES:

White bread, crusts removed

Crab Salad (see page 144)

Spread trimmed bread with prepared crab salad. Slice bread diagonally to make four triangles.

CUCUMBER SANDWICHES:

White bread, cut with 2–inch biscuit cutter
Cream Cheese Butter (see page 53)

Cucumbers, peeled and sliced
Fresh dill

Spread bread rounds with cream cheese butter. Place a thin slice of cucumber on top. Garnish with a sprig of fresh dill.

TOMATO SANDWICHES:

White bread, cut with 2–inch biscuit cutter
Cream Cheese Butter (see page 53)

Cherry tomatoes, washed and sliced
Parsley

Spread bread rounds with cream cheese butter. Place a thin slice of tomato on top. Garnish with a sprig of fresh parsley.

Bacon Crisps

Fat–free Parmesan cheese
Reduced fat Waverly wafers

Oscar Mayer Bacon, cut into fourths

Heap cheese on top of each cracker. Place bacon over cheese. Place on broiler pan rack. Bake at 200° for 2 to 2½ hours. Drain on paper towels. Eat hot or cold.

Artichoke Dip

1 (14–ounce) can artichoke
   hearts, drained
½ cup fat–free Parmesan cheese
½ cup fat–free mozzarella
   cheese

½ teaspoon garlic powder
¼ teaspoon salt
1 cup Weight Watcher's Fat
   Free Whipped Dressing

Break up artichoke hearts with fork and mix with remaining ingredients. Bake in a Pam–sprayed casserole dish at 350° for 15–20 minutes or until golden brown. Serve warm with assorted low–fat crackers.

Asparagus Rolls

Fat–free bread, crusts removed
Ultra Promise 70% Less Fat
Asparagus spears

Fat–free Parmesan cheese
Butter salt
Butter flavor Pam spray

With a rolling pin, flatten bread slice. Spread with thin layer of Promise. Place asparagus spear on top and roll up in bread. Spray with Pam spray, roll in cheese; sprinkle with butter salt. Place on Pam–sprayed cookie sheet. Cook at 325° until golden; turn and continue cooking until golden. Serve hot.

Cheese Bites

¼ cup green onions, thinly
   sliced
2 tablespoons pimento, drained
   and chopped
2 teaspoons capers, drained
   and chopped

2 cups fat–free Cheddar cheese,
   grated
½ cup Weight Watcher's Fat
   Free Whipped Dressing
6 English muffins, halved
Fat-free Parmesan cheese
Garlic powder

Combine onions, pimento, capers, cheese and whipped dressing. Spread evenly over muffin halves. Sprinkle with Parmesan cheese and garlic powder. Bake at 350° for 15 to 20 minutes. Cut muffin halves into quarters. Serve warm.

Bacon Wrapped Dates

1 (8–ounce) package pitted dates   Oscar Mayer Bacon

Wrap each date with one fourth of a strip of bacon and skewer with toothpick. Bake at 350° for 12 to 15 minutes or until bacon is crisp. Drain on paper towels. Serve hot. Makes approximately 3 dozen.

Blue Cheese Spread

1 (8–ounce) package fat–free
   cream cheese
1 teaspoon onion, grated
½ teaspoon Worcestershire sauce

¼ teaspoon salt
3 tablespoons fat–free blue
   cheese salad dressing

Beat cream cheese. Add remaining ingredients and mix well. Best if made ahead of time so that flavors can blend. Serve with assorted low–fat crackers.

Cheese and Crabmeat Dip

1 teaspoon garlic salt
1 (8–ounce) package fat–free
   cream cheese, softened
½ pint fat–free sour cream

1 teaspoon curry powder
1 package Louis Kemp
   imitation crabmeat

Beat cream cheese until smooth. Add remaining ingredients, mixing well. Serve with assorted low–fat crackers.

Fresh Fruit Dip

1 (7–ounce) jar marshmallow
   creme

1 (8–ounce) package fat–free
   cream cheese

Mix thoroughly and serve with fresh fruits such as apples, strawberries, peaches, etc.

Cheesy Diamonds

PASTRY:

1½ cups all–purpose flour
¾ teaspoon salt
¼ teaspoon paprika

½ cup Ultra Promise 70% Less Fat
½ cup fat–free sour cream

For pastry, mix together flour, salt and paprika. Cut in Ultra Promise. Add sour cream and mix until well blended. Cover and chill at least 15 minutes before using.

FILLING:

¾ cup water chestnuts, finely chopped
¾ cup pimento, chopped
¾ cup fat–free Cheddar cheese, shredded

2 tablespoons Weight Watcher's Fat Free Whipped Dressing
3 green onions, chopped

While dough is chilling assemble filling ingredients. Mix together all ingredients. Divide dough in half. Roll each half to a rectangle 8x15–inch; then cut two 4–inch strips. Spread center of each strip with filling. Fold edges over to enclose it completely, moistening edges which overlap so they will seal. Invert onto a Pam–sprayed baking sheet, seam side down. Bake at 400° for about 10 minutes. Cool and cut in diagonal slices to make diamonds. Makes about 3 dozen.

Chip Dip

1 (8–ounce) package fat–free cream cheese
5 tablespoons Weight Watcher's Fat Free Whipped Dressing

1½ tablespoons Worcestershire sauce
2 tablespoons onion, grated
Garlic salt to taste
¼ teaspoon Tabasco
Pinch of white pepper

Beat cream cheese until smooth. Add remaining ingredients. Best if made ahead so that flavors can blend. Serve with low–fat potato chips.

Chive Cheese Balls

4 ounces fat–free cream cheese
1 teaspoon garlic powder
2 teaspoons dried chives or 1
  tablespoon plus 1 teaspoon
  fresh chives

1 package refrigerated biscuits
  (1 fat gram or less per biscuit)

Mix first 3 ingredients well. Put back into refrigerator until thoroughly chilled so mixture can be handled easier. Separate biscuits; flatten and cut in half. Put small amount of cheese mixture in center of each piece of dough. Fold dough around mixture, forming a ball. Place on a Pam–sprayed cookie sheet. Bake at 350° for 8 minutes or until golden brown. Serve hot.

Chutney Cheese Ball

6 ounces fat–free Cheddar
  cheese, shredded
1 (8–ounce) package fat–free
  cream cheese, softened
¾ teaspoon curry powder
3 tablespoons dry sherry

¼ teaspoon salt
½ teaspoon parsley flakes
1½ to 2 cups chutney
1½ to 2 cups green onion,
  finely chopped

In a bowl, beat cream cheese. Then add Cheddar cheese, curry, sherry, salt and parsley. Shape mixture into a ball or rectangle. Chill overnight. To serve, top with chutney and sprinkle with green onions. Serve with assorted low–fat crackers.

Crab Petites

1 package large flour tortillas
⅓ cup Weight Watcher's Fat
  Free Whipped Dressing
2 tablespoons green onions,
  chopped

¼ cup red peppers, finely
  chopped
1 cup fat–free Cheddar cheese,
  shredded
1 (5–ounce) can crabmeat

Combine all ingredients, excluding tortillas; mix well. Spread mixture thinly over tortillas and roll them up. Wrap, individually, in plastic wrap. Refrigerate overnight. Slice and serve with cocktail sauce.

Crabmeat Dip

1 (8–ounce) package Louis Kemp imitation crab, processed in food processor
⅔ cup fat–free sour cream
1 tablespoon horseradish or to taste
½ teaspoon pepper
2 tablespoons fat–free Italian dressing
Salt to taste

Mix all ingredients together. Best if made ahead so that flavors can blend. Serve with assorted low–fat crackers.

Crisp Cheese Wafers

2 ounces Kroger Lite Classics Sharp Cheddar cheese, shredded
6 ounces fat–free Cheddar cheese, shredded
8 tablespoons Ultra Promise 70% Less Fat
1 cup flour
½ teaspoon salt
½ teaspoon red pepper
¼ teaspoon paprika
1 cup Rice Krispies

Mix cheese with Ultra Promise 70% Less Fat. Add dry ingredients. Fold in Rice Krispies. Roll into balls and flatten into small wafers with a fork. Bake on Pam–sprayed cookie sheet at 350° for 12 minutes. Makes about 4 dozen.

Curry Chicken Ball

4 ounces fat–free cream cheese
2 tablespoons Weight Watcher's Fat Free Whipped Dressing
1 cup chicken breast, finely chopped or processed in food processor
1 cup dates, chopped
1 teaspoon sugar
1 tablespoon chutney
½ teaspoon salt
2 teaspoons curry powder
Parsley

Mix cream cheese and whipped dressing. Add chicken, dates, sugar, chutney, salt and curry powder. Chill. Before serving, sprinkle with parsley flakes. Serve with assorted low–fat and fat–free crackers.

Curry Dip I

1 cup Weight Watcher's Fat
  Free Whipped Dressing
1 teaspoon curry powder
¼ teaspoon garlic powder

1 teaspoon tarragon vinegar
1 teaspoon onion powder
1 teaspoon horseradish
Salt to taste

Combine all ingredients. Best if made ahead so that flavors can blend. Chill. Serve with low–fat crackers or raw vegetables.

Curry Dip II

1 cup Weight Watcher's Fat
  Free Whipped Dressing
1 tablespoon ketchup
1½ teaspoons Worcestershire
  sauce
2 tablespoons onion, grated

1 teaspoon curry powder
  or to taste
½ teaspoon Tabasco
Salt to taste
1 teaspoon white wine

Mix all ingredients together. Best if made ahead so that flavors can blend. Serve with fresh, raw vegetables.

Garden Mold

2 envelopes unflavored gelatin
1 pint Weight Watcher's Fat
  Free Whipped Dressing
1 teaspoon salt
¼ teaspoon white pepper

2 tomatoes, peeled and finely
  chopped
1 small onion, finely chopped
1 cup celery, finely chopped
1 bell pepper, finely chopped
1 cucumber, finely chopped

Dissolve gelatin in ¼ cup cold water. Add ¼ cup boiling water and mix well. Add whipped dressing, salt and pepper and mix well. Add chopped vegetables and mix. Coat a 6–cup mold ring with whipped dressing. Pour mixture into mold, cover with plastic wrap and re-frigerate at least 6 to 8 hours. Serve with crackers.

Garlic Grilled Cheese

2 slices lowfat bread
1 slice Borden's Free Cheese
   Singles
Garlic powder

I Can't Believe It's Not Butter
   Spray
Kraft Parmesan fat-free cheese

Place cheese between bread slices. Sprinkle garlic on top slice of bread. Spray with Butter Spray. Toast, top only, in toaster oven. When golden, remove and repeat with garlic and Butter Spray. Sprinkle with Parmesan cheese. Toast until golden brown. Serve hot with soup, fruit salads, etc.

Goat Cheese Spread

1 (8–ounce) package fat–free
   cream cheese
8 ounces goat cheese

2 teaspoons fresh thyme leaves,
   finely chopped
3 sweet red peppers
Parsley

Combine first 3 ingredients, blending until smooth. Press mixture into a mold lined with plastic wrap and chill. Roast peppers over gas flame or under broiler, turning until the skins are charred all over. Place peppers in a bowl and cover tightly and set aside for 20 minutes. Halve the peppers and remove cores, peel off skin. Cut peppers into 1–inch strips and place in food processor; pulse 3 or 4 times. Unmold chilled cheese mixture; top with red pepper puree. Garnish with parsley. Serve with crostini or Melba toast.

Goat Cheese Tomato Sauce

1 (14½–ounce) can DelMonte
   fresh cut diced tomatoes
Salt and pepper to taste

¾ teaspoon basil
2 tablespoons goat cheese

Combine first 3 ingredients in a small saucepan. Cover. Bring to a boil and gently boil for about 30 minutes or until tomatoes are reduced to about one half. Add goat cheese and stir until melted. May be served over fettuccine.

17

Goat Cheese Puffs

2 tablespoons Ultra Promise
  70% Less Fat
8 tablespoons goat cheese
2 teaspoons basil
3 tablespoons dried tomatoes,
  finely chopped

1½ cups fat–free mozzarella
  cheese, shredded
1 cup flour
1 egg white
1 tablespoon water

Cream together Ultra Promise 70% Less Fat, goat cheese, basil and tomatoes. Add mozzarella cheese, mixing well. Add flour. Shape into 1–inch balls. Brush with egg white mixed with water. Bake on Pam–sprayed cooking sheet at 350° for 10 minutes. Makes approximately 30.

VARIATION: Replace basil with 2 teaspoons tarragon.

Hot Goat Cheese Puffs

2 tablespoons Ultra Promise
  70% Less Fat
8 tablespoons goat cheese
1½ tablespoons dried tomatoes,
  chopped extra fine

¾ cup fat–free mozzarella
  cheese, shredded
½ cup flour
1 teaspoon basil or tarragon

Cream Ultra Promise with cheeses. Add remaining ingredients; mix well. Roll into 1–inch balls. Bake on Pam–sprayed cookie sheet at 350° for 10 to 12 minutes.

Honey Mustard Vegetable Dip

½ cup Weight Watcher's Fat
  Free Whipped Dressing

2 tablespoons Dijon mustard
1 tablespoon honey

Mix together and serve with assorted raw vegetables.

Hot Shrimp Melts

2 tablespoons onion, chopped
1 tablespoon Ultra Promise
  70% Less Fat
1½ tablespoons flour
1 teaspoon dry mustard
1 cup skim milk

6 ounces shrimp (canned or
  frozen; if frozen, thoroughly
  thaw and dry on paper towels)
4 English muffins, halved
1 cup fat–free Cheddar cheese,
  shredded

Sauté onions in a non–stick Pam–sprayed skillet. In a separate bowl, mix Ultra Promise, flour, dry mustard and 5 tablespoons milk until all lumps are gone. Stir in remaining milk and add to onions. Cook until thickened, stirring constantly. Stir in shrimp; remove from heat. Spoon shrimp mixture onto muffins. Top with cheese. Broil until bubbly. Cut into quarters.

Italian Cheese Puffs

½ cup Ultra Promise 70% Less
  Fat
2 cups fat–free mozzarella
  cheese, shredded
1 cup flour

¼ teaspoon paprika
1 to 2 teaspoons Italian
  seasoning
1 egg white
1 tablespoon water

Cream Ultra Promise with cheese. Add flour, paprika and seasoning. Shape into 1–inch balls. Mix egg white and water. Brush puffs with egg white mixture. Bake on a Pam–sprayed cooking sheet at 350° for 10 minutes. Makes 30 to 36.

Katie's Cheese Straws

1 pound Kroger Sensible
  Indulgence sharp Cheddar
  cheese, shredded
2 cups flour

½ teaspoon salt
1½ teaspoons cayenne pepper
½ cup Ultra Promise 70% Less
  Fat

Sift flour, salt and pepper together. Cream cheese and Ultra Promise; gradually add dry ingredients. Place between wax paper and roll ¼–inch thickness. Cut into strips. Bake on a Pam–sprayed cookie sheet at 400° for 10 minutes. Do not overbake.

19

Kathy's Chutney Cheese Ball

1 (8–ounce) package fat–free
cream cheese
1 tablespoon parsley flakes
2 tablespoons Weight
Watcher's Fat Free Whipped
Dressing
¼ teaspoon cayenne pepper
¼ teaspoon garlic powder

Salt to taste
8 ounces fat–free Cheddar
cheese, shredded
1 jar Major Grey Chutney
5 slices Oscar Mayer bacon,
fried crisp, well drained and
crumbled

Beat cream cheese to soften. Add parsley, whipped dressing, pepper, garlic and salt; mix well. Add Cheddar cheese. Mold into a square and refrigerate overnight. To serve, remove from container, top with chutney and crumbled bacon. Serve with assorted low–fat crackers.

Kathy's Layered Crabmeat Surprise

2 (8–ounce) packages fat–free
cream cheese, softened
1 large bunch green onions,
chopped
3 ribs celery, finely chopped
2 medium tomatoes, chopped
and drained

6 to 8 ounces fat–free
mozzarella cheese, shredded
6 to 8 ounces fat–free Parmesan
cheese
2½ packages Louis Kemp's
imitation or 24 ounces fresh
crabmeat or shrimp
2 bottles chili sauce

Layer first 6 ingredients in a serving dish in order given. Chop crabmeat (or shrimp). Divide crabmeat. Layer half of crabmeat on top of Parmesan cheese. Pour chili sauce over crabmeat. Top with remaining crabmeat. Chill. Serve with assorted low–fat or fat–free crackers.

Hot Crabmeat Canapes

1 (8–ounce) package Louis
   Kemp imitation crabmeat,
   finely diced
6 tablespoons Weight
   Watcher's Fat Free Whipped
   Dressing

Salt to taste
1 tablespoon onion, grated
1 teaspoon lemon juice
½ cup fat–free Parmesan cheese
Small rounds of white bread
Paprika

Mix together first 6 ingredients. Pile the mixture on bread rounds. Sprinkle with paprika. Place under the broiler until golden brown. Makes about 3 dozen.

Marinated Mushrooms

1 pound fresh mushrooms,
   washed and drained
⅓ cup red wine vinegar
⅓ cup vinaigrette fat–free
   dressing
1 teaspoon dry mustard

1½ teaspoons brown sugar
2 teaspoons dried parsley
1 teaspoon salt
⅛ teaspoon pepper
1 small onion, diced

Heat all ingredients, except mushrooms, to boiling. Cook 5 minutes. Remove from heat, pour over mushrooms. Cool. Refrigerate for several hours or overnight.

Mexican Tortilla Dip

1 (#2) can black beans, rinsed
   and drained
1 (#2) can whole kernel corn,
   drained
1 (#2) can stewed tomatoes,
   drained and reserving half of
   liquid

¼ cup taco seasoning mix
6 to 8 green onions, with stems,
   coarsely chopped
Juice of 1 lime

Combine all ingredients and mix well. Keep refrigerated. Serve with low–fat tortilla chips.

Lobster Mousse

1 can Campbell's tomato soup
1 (8–ounce) package fat–free
   cream cheese
1 cup celery, very finely
   chopped
½ cup green pepper, very
   finely chopped
2 tablespoons onion, grated
2 envelopes unflavored gelatin

1 cup cold water
1 (8–ounce) package Louis
   Kemp imitation lobster,
   processed in food processor
   or very finely chopped
Salt and white pepper to taste
Basil and/or paprika for
   garnish

Heat soup to boiling. Soften gelatin in water and add to hot soup. Beat until dissolved. Cut cheese in small cubes. Gradually add cheese to soup. Beat with mixer until smooth. Add remaining ingredients; mix well. Pour into Pam–sprayed mold. Garnish with basil and/or paprika. Serve with assorted low–fat crackers.

Lobster Pâté with Cherry Tomatoes

3 to 4 celery ribs, finely
   chopped
2 green onions, finely chopped
1 teaspoon Worcestershire
   sauce
Juice of 1 lemon
6 ounces fat–free cream cheese

¼ cup Weight Watcher's Fat
   Free Whipped Dressing
¾ teaspoon white pepper
Salt to taste
1 teaspoon Tabasco
Cherry tomatoes

Mix together all ingredients excluding tomatoes. Wash and core tomatoes. Fill tomatoes with lobster mixture. Serve chilled with assorted low–fat crackers.

Onion Parmesan Bake

3 cups Vidalia onions, diced
1 cup Weight Watcher's Fat
  Free Whipped Dressing

1 cup fat–free Parmesan cheese

In a hot Pam–sprayed skillet, sauté onions. Mix with whipped dressing and cheese. Place in a Pam–sprayed casserole dish. Bake at 350° for 30 minutes or until golden. Serve hot with low–fat or fat–free crackers.

Parmesan Cheese Straws

1¼ cups fat–free Parmesan
  cheese
1 cup flour
8 tablespoons Ultra Promise
  70% Less Fat, room
  temperature
¾ teaspoon marjoram

¾ teaspoon oregano
¾ teaspoon basil
¼ teaspoon cayenne pepper or
  to taste
½ teaspoon Worcestershire
  sauce
3 tablespoons dry white wine

Blend cheese, flour, Ultra Promise and seasonings to a coarse meal. Add Worcestershire and wine to form a ball. Divide dough and roll into a log 1 inch in diameter. Wrap in plastic wrap and chill for 1 hour. Cut into 1½–inch long pieces. Cut each lengthwise into fourths. Place on a Pam–sprayed cooking sheet. Flatten using a fork. Bake at 400° for 10 minutes. Serve fresh from the oven. Makes 48.

Bacon–Wrapped Hors D'oeuvres

2 (10–ounce) cans whole water
  chestnuts

1 bottle soy sauce
½ pound Oscar Mayer bacon

Marinate water chestnuts in soy sauce for at least two hours. Wrap each in ⅓ strip bacon. Secure with toothpicks. Bake at 400° for 10 to 15 minutes or until bacon is crisp. Serve hot. Can be made ahead of time and refrigerated until time to serve.

Oven–Baked Fried Cheese

1 Egg Beater
½ envelope Shake–N–Bake
  Country Mild for chicken
Garlic powder to taste

Fat–free Parmesan cheese
6 ounces Alpine Lace Fat Free
  mozzarella block cheese
  cut ½–inch thick

Mix Shake–N–Bake and garlic. Dip cheese into Egg Beater. Roll in Shake–N–Bake mixture then roll in Parmesan cheese. Broil on second shelf of oven for about 2 minutes until golden brown and cheese swells.

VARIATIONS: Alpine Lace Fat Free Cheddar cheese may be substituted for the mozzarella cheese.

Shake–N–Bake Hot and Spicy for Chicken may be substituted for the Shake–N–Bake Country Mild for Chicken.

Add 1 tablespoon dried basil to Shake–N–Bake Country Mild for Chicken.

Oyster Delight

3 jars oysters, drained
3 ribs celery, chopped
¼ cup Fleischmann's Fat Free
  Squeezable Spread
1 large onion, chopped
1½ cups evaporated skimmed
  milk
½ cup mushrooms, sliced
1 tablespoon Worcestershire
  sauce

2 teaspoons celery salt
3 tablespoons fresh lemon
  juice
¾ teaspoon Tabasco
Pinch of white pepper
Salt to taste
2 tablespoons cornstarch
2 tablespoons evaporated
  skimmed milk

Cut oysters in small pieces. Boil celery until tender. Sauté onions in a Pam–sprayed non–stick skillet. Add oysters, celery, milk and all other ingredients. Start tasting until tangy. Add more Tabasco, lemon juice or Worcestershire, if you desire. Stir and keep tasting; this must be seasoned to taste. Cook for 20 minutes over low heat. Add 2 tablespoons cornstarch mixed with 2 tablespoons milk to thicken. Serve in chafing dish with Melba rounds.

Pepper Pie

2 (4.5–ounce) cans green chilies
4 ounces Kroger Lite Classics
   Sharp Cheddar cheese,
   shredded

½ cup fat–free Cheddar cheese,
   shredded
4 Egg Beaters
Salt and white pepper to taste

Drain chilies and line bottom and sides of a 9–inch pie plate. Press grated cheese in plate over chilies. Beat Egg Beaters with salt and pepper. Pour over cheese. Bake at 350° for 20 minutes. Slice into small wedges. Serve hot.

Pickled Shrimp

1¾ cups fat–free Italian
   dressing
1 teaspoon black pepper
2 teaspoons horseradish
2 tablespoons prepared
   mustard

2 stalks celery, chopped
2 drops red food coloring
1 pound shrimp, cooked,
   deveined and peeled

In mixing bowl, combine first 6 ingredients. Pour over prepared shrimp. Cover and refrigerate 24 hours before serving.

Pineapple Cheese Ball

2 (8–ounce) packages fat–free
   cream cheese, softened
1 (8½–ounce) can crushed
   pineapple, well–drained
¼ cup green pepper, finely
   chopped

2 tablespoons onion, finely
   chopped
1 tablespoon seasoned salt
1 teaspoon sugar
4 teaspoons pineapple
   preserves

Whip cream cheese with mixer to soften. Add remaining ingredients, stirring well. Shape into a ball and refrigerate. Serve with low–fat crackers.

Potpourri Dip

1 can green chilies, chopped
2 cups tomatoes, peeled and
  finely chopped
½ teaspoon wine vinegar

Dash of Tabasco
3 green onions, finely chopped
Dash of garlic
Salt to taste

Mix and chill. Serve with low–fat tortilla chips.

Quick Refried Beans

4 green onions, thinly sliced
1 (4–ounce) can green chilies
1 (16–ounce) can fat–free
  refried beans
1 tablespoon ground cumin

¾ teaspoon garlic powder
¼ teaspoon cayenne pepper
1½ cups fat–free Cheddar
  cheese, shredded

Briefly sauté green onions in Pam–sprayed skillet. Combine remaining ingredients. May be heated in 350° oven for 15 minutes or served cold. Serve with low–fat tortilla chips.

Salmon Pâté

1 (6–ounce) can Chicken of the
  Sea (2 fat grams per serving)
  salmon
1 (8–ounce) package fat–free
  cream cheese, softened
3 tablespoons onions, finely
  chopped

2 tablespoons chili sauce
4 tablespoons fresh parsley,
  chopped and divided
2 tablespoons horseradish
2 dashes Tabasco, optional

Combine all ingredients except 2 tablespoons parsley. Form into log or ball; chill overnight. Sprinkle with remaining parsley. Serve with lowfat crackers.

"Sausage" Balls

1½ cups Pioneer low–fat
  biscuit mix
1 pound fat–free Cheddar
  cheese or mozzarella cheese
  or ½ pound each

1 pound Country Turkey
  Sausage (see page 218)

Combine all ingredients until dough sticks together. Roll into 1½–
inch balls. Bake at 350° for 15 minutes. Makes 75 balls.

Shrimp Appetizers

1 (8–ounce) package fat–free
  cream cheese
4 tablespoons Weight
  Watcher's Fat Free Whipped
  Dressing
2 tablespoons ketchup
2 teaspoons prepared mustard
½ teaspoon garlic salt or to
  taste

Dash celery salt
2 cups fresh or frozen shrimp,
  cooked and finely chopped
½ cup celery, finely chopped
2 teaspoons onion, grated
Athen's Mini Fillo Dough
  Shells

In a small mixing bowl, blend first 6 ingredients until smooth. Stir in
shrimp, celery and onion. Fill Fillo Shells with shrimp mixture.

Shrimp Dijon

Shrimp, cooked, peeled,
  deveined and chilled

Dijon Basil Vinaigrette
  (see page 66)
Lettuce

Place shrimp on lettuce leaf. Top with dressing. Serve cold.

Shrimp Dip

1 (8–ounce) package fat–free
   cream cheese
5 ounces cooked shrimp,
   deveined and peeled

4 tablespoons Weight
   Watcher's Fat Free Whipped
   Dressing
1 teaspoon seasoning salt
2 teaspoons onion, chopped

Mix all ingredients in blender. Chill. Best if made ahead so that flavors can blend. Serve with assorted low fat crackers.

Shrimp Hors D'oeuvres

1 pound shrimp, cooked and
   peeled
1 onion, chopped
2 cups Weight Watcher's Fat
   Free Whipped Dressing

2 cups fat–free Parmesan
   cheese
Parsley
Salt to taste

Put shrimp through food processor or chop fine. Mix all ingredients. Serve on white or whole wheat bread rounds.

Shrimp Mold

1 envelope unflavored gelatin
½ cup cold water
6 ounces fresh or frozen
   shrimp, finely chopped
2 tablespoons fresh lemon
   juice
¼ teaspoon Tabasco

¾ cup Weight Watcher's Fat
   Free Whipped Dressing
1 teaspoon dried minced onion
½ cup celery, finely diced
¼ cup green pepper, finely
   diced

Sprinkle gelatin in cold water. Place over boiling water and stir until gelatin is dissolved. Add lemon juice and Tabasco. Let cool. Gradually add gelatin mixture to whipped dressing. Stir until blended. Mix in remaining ingredients. Turn into Pam–sprayed large mold or small individual molds. Chill until firm.

Shrimp Spread

6 ounces fat–free cream cheese
1 teaspoon onion, grated
1 teaspoon lemon juice
½ teaspoon Worcestershire
 sauce
½ pound cooked, deveined
 shrimp
½ cup Weight Watcher's Fat
 Free Whipped Dressing
Salt and pepper to taste

Beat cream cheese. Add onion, lemon juice and Worcestershire sauce. Chop shrimp in food processor. Add to cream cheese mixture. Add remaining ingredients and mix well. Best if made ahead so that flavors can blend.

Spicy Carolina Crabmeat

2 (8–ounce) packages fat–free
 cream cheese, room
 temperature
⅛ teaspoon white pepper
⅓ cup onion, minced
1 tablespoon Worcestershire
 sauce
1 tablespoon Weight Watcher's
 Fat Free Whipped Dressing
½ teaspoon garlic powder
1 pound Louis Kemp imitation
 crabmeat, processed in food
 processor
1 (12–ounce) bottle chili sauce
Parsley to garnish

Mix cream cheese until soft. Add next 5 ingredients. Shape mixture into a square. Chill until set. Before serving, spread crabmeat over cheese mixture. Cover with chili sauce. Garnish with fresh parsley. (Make cream cheese mixture a day ahead so that flavors can blend.)

Tuna Spread

1 (6–ounce) can water–packed
 tuna, drained
1 envelope instant onion soup
1 cup fat–free sour cream
4 teaspoons prepared
 horseradish

Mix all ingredients well. Let chill for several hours before serving. Serve with low–fat or fat–free crackers or low–fat potato chips.

Stuffed Shrimp

1½ pounds large shrimp
½ pound crabmeat
⅓ cup onion, finely chopped
¼ cup green pepper, finely
  chopped
2 tablespoons flour
2 tablespoons Fleischmann's
  Fat Free Squeezable Spread
¾ teaspoon salt
⅛ teaspoon pepper

1 cup skim milk
1 teaspoon dry sherry
1 teaspoon dry mustard
2 tablespoons Weight
  Watcher's Fat Free Whipped
  Dressing
¼ cup fat–free Parmesan cheese
I Can't Believe It's Not Butter
  Spray
Paprika

Wash shrimp, shell and devein. Make a cut lengthwise down the back of each shrimp. Drain crabmeat and remove any shell. Sauté onion and green pepper in a non–stick Pam–sprayed skillet. Blend flour, Fleischmann's, salt, pepper and milk. Whisk until all lumps are removed. Cook until thickened, stirring constantly. Add sherry, mustard, whipped dressing and crabmeat; mix well. Stuff shrimp with crabmeat mixture. Sprinkle with Parmesan cheese. Spray with Butter Spray. Sprinkle with paprika. Bake at 350° for 12 to 15 minutes.

Quick Mini Pizzas

1 (6–ounce) can tomato paste
1 cup water
1 teaspoon oregano
¼ teaspoon sugar
½ teaspoon garlic
Salt to taste

Fat–free Parmesan cheese
6 English muffins, split,
  toasted
2 cups fat–free mozzarella
  cheese, shredded

Combine first 6 ingredients. Spread on toasted muffins, sprinkle with Parmesan cheese. Top with mozzarella cheese. May be eaten as is or with desired Canadian bacon, green pepper, mushrooms, etc.

Tuna Mold

1 envelope unflavored gelatin
½ cup cold water
1 can water–packed tuna, drained
2 tablespoons fresh lemon juice
¼ teaspoon Tabasco

¾ cup Weight Watcher's Fat Free Whipped Dressing
1 teaspoon dried minced onion
½ cup celery, finely chopped
¼ cup green pepper, finely chopped

Sprinkle gelatin in cold water. Place over boiling water and stir until gelatin is dissolved. Add lemon juice and Tabasco. Let cool. Gradually add gelatin mixture to whipped dressing. Stir until blended. Mix in remaining ingredients. Pour into a Pam–sprayed large mold or small individual molds. Chill until firm.

Vegetable Dip

1 cup Weight Watcher's Fat Free Whipped Dressing
½ teaspoon fresh lemon juice
¼ teaspoon salt
¼ teaspoon paprika
1 teaspoon dried minced onion

1 teaspoon Greek Seasoning
1 teaspoon dried chives
⅛ teaspoon curry powder
½ teaspoon Worcestershire sauce
½ cup fat–free sour cream

Mix all ingredients together. Chill at least 2 hours before serving. Serve with raw celery, carrots, cauliflower and broccoli.

Vegetables Canapes

1 (8–ounce) package fat–free cream cheese
1 envelope Italian dressing mix
¼ cup Dijon mustard

¾ cup fat–free sour cream
1 teaspoon dried parsley
Assorted fresh vegetables

Combine all ingredients, except vegetables, in food processor; process until smooth. Chill until slightly firm. Spoon or pipe with pastry tube onto vegetables.

Vidalia Onion Dip

2 cups Weight Watcher's Fat
  Free Whipped Dressing
2 cups fat–free mozzarella
  cheese, shredded

3 cups Vidalia onions, chopped
1 (8–ounce) can sliced water
  chestnuts, drained
Pinch of white pepper

Combine all ingredients in a Pam–sprayed 2–quart baking dish. Bake at 350° for 30 minutes. Serve with Melba rounds or low–fat crackers.

Party Franks

1 pound fat–free frankfurters
1 (10–ounce) jar currant jelly

½ cup mustard
1 tablespoon horseradish

Heat jelly, mustard and horseradish until melted. Boil frankfurters until thoroughly heated. Cut into 1–inch pieces. Add to jelly mixture. Heat and serve.

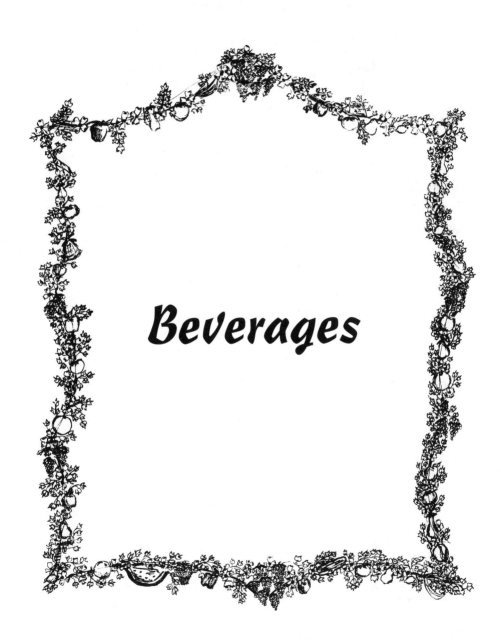

Beverages

Apple–Orange Hot Cider

1 gallon apple cider
1 cup sugar
3 cups orange juice
1 (6–ounce) can frozen
lemonade concentrate,
thawed

1 teaspoon whole allspice
(optional)
2 teaspoons whole cloves
2 sticks cinnamon

Mix together first 4 ingredients, stirring to dissolve sugar. Remove 3 cups of cider mixture into a small saucepan. Add allspice, cloves and cinnamon; bring to a boil. Remove from heat, cover and let steep until cool. Strain and return to cider mixture. Keep refrigerated until needed. Serve hot.

Apple–Wine Punch

3 cups apple cider
¼ cup sugar
3 cinnamon sticks

6 whole cloves
1 bottle dry white wine
2 tablespoons lemon juice

In saucepan combine first 4 ingredients and bring to a boil. Stir to dissolve sugar. Simmer, uncovered, for 15 minutes. Strain. Add wine and lemon juice. Heat through, but do not boil. Serve hot in mugs.

Banana Whiz

2 ripened bananas
2 cups cold skim milk

1 cup vanilla fat–free ice cream
1¼ teaspoons vanilla

Mash bananas. Add all ingredients in blender and process until smooth.

Betty's Dessert Coffee

4 cups coffee   ½ teaspoon ground cinnamon

Per 4 cups of coffee add ½ teaspoon of cinnamon. Perk or prepare as directed.

Brunch Champagne Punch

1 (6–ounce) can frozen   ½ cup Triple Sec liqueur
   lemonade concentrate,   ¼ cup orange juice
   thawed   1 bottle champagne, chilled
2½ cups water, divided

Mix half the concentrate and 1½ cups water; freeze into ice cubes. At serving time, combine liqueur, orange juice, remaining concentrate and 1 cup water in a 2–quart pitcher. Add lemonade cubes. Slowly pour in champagne; stir gently and serve immediately.

Brunch Punch

3 quarts pineapple juice   2½ cups sugar
1½ cups fresh lemon juice   4 (1–pint) bottles ginger ale,
3 cups orange juice   chilled
½ cup fresh lime juice

Combine first 5 ingredients; mix well. Chill. Just before serving add chilled ginger ale.

Cape Cod Cider Punch

Juice of 3 oranges   ¼ cup maraschino cherries
Juice of 1 lemon   1 quart apple cider
                               Sugar to taste

Mix together first 4 ingredients. Taste for sweetness and add sugar according to taste. Refrigerate.

Carol's Texas Tea

7 regular sized tea bags
15 sprigs fresh mint
1 quart boiling water
1 cup sugar

1 large can frozen lemonade
4 cans water
1½ cups pineapple juice

Place first 3 ingredients in pan and bring to boil. Remove from heat; cover and steep for 30 minutes. Drain mixture; add sugar and stir until dissolved. Add remaining ingredients and stir. May be served hot or cold.

Champagne Punch

2 (16–ounce) cans pitted dark
   sweet cherries, drained,
   reserving 2 tablespoons juice
1 (12–ounce) can pineapple
   juice

½ cup brandy
¼ cup lemon juice
1 tablespoon sugar
2 bottles champagne, chilled

Drain cherries, reserving 2 tablespoons juice. Combine drained cherries, pineapple juice, brandy, lemon juice, sugar and reserved cherry juice. Chill thoroughly to blend flavors. Just before serving, pour into punch bowl. Carefully add champagne, pouring down side of bowl. Gently stir; serve immediately.

Christmas Boiled Custard

2 (3.4–ounce) packages vanilla
   instant pudding
1 can fat–free Eagle Brand milk

¼ cup sugar
½ gallon skim milk

Mix together and chill. Will thicken as it chills. May be thinned with skim milk.

Cinnamon Coffee Punch

8 cinnamon sticks
1 gallon hot, strong coffee
2 cups Dream Whip, prepared,
 or Cool Whip Free

4 teaspoons vanilla
2 quarts fat–free vanilla ice
 cream
¼ cup sugar

Add cinnamon sticks to hot coffee. Set aside until cold; remove cinnamon. Add vanilla, ice cream and sugar. Fold in Dream Whip or Cool Whip.

Coffee Punch Surprise

3½ cups skim milk
½ cup triple–strength coffee,
 chilled
3 tablespoons sugar

1 teaspoon orange extract
Orange sherbet
Mandarin oranges, drained, for
 garnish

Combine first 4 ingredients in punch bowl. Top with scoops of sherbet and mandarin oranges.

Company Spiced Cider

1 gallon apple cider
½ cup brown sugar
1 tablespoon sugar
2 lemons, sliced

2 oranges, sliced
8 whole cloves, studded in fruit
 slices
4 cinnamon sticks

Combine all ingredients in a saucepan. Bring to a boil; reduce heat and simmer for 10 minutes.

Cranberry Fruit Tea

4 quarts water
3 cups sugar
2 (6–ounce) cans frozen lemon
   juice

1 quart apple juice
2 quarts cranberry juice
1 pint orange juice
1 pint strong black tea

Mix water and sugar in large saucepan; bring to a boil. Boil for 3 minutes. Set aside to cool. Combine juices, tea and sugar syrup. Mix well. Chill before serving.

Creamy Fruit Punch

2½ cups pineapple juice,
   chilled
½ cup pineapple tidbits,
   drained

1 pint raspberry sherbet
1 pint fat–free vanilla ice cream
1 (12–ounce) bottle sparkling
   water, chilled

Combine juice, pineapple, sherbet and half of ice cream, beating until smooth. Add sparkling water. Spoon remaining ice cream into punch; serve immediately.

Creamy Peach Shake

1 pint fat–free vanilla ice
   cream, softened
¾ cup canned sliced peaches,
   drained and chilled

¾ cup unsweetened pineapple
   juice, chilled
1 cup skim milk, chilled
Fresh mint for garnish

Place ice cream, peaches and pineapple juice in blender. Process on high until smooth. Add milk and vanilla. Process again. Pour into tall glasses and garnish with fresh mint.

Daiquiri Party Punch

2 (6–ounce) cans frozen
   limeade concentrate, thawed
1 (6–ounce) can frozen
   lemonade concentrate,
   thawed
1 (6–ounce) can frozen orange
   juice concentrate, thawed

8 cups water
1 ⅕ quart rum
4 cups carbonated water,
   chilled
4 slices each of lemon, lime
   and orange

Combine concentrates with water; chill. To serve, combine rum with punch in punch bowl. Carefully pour in carbonated water. Float fruit slices on top.

Dessert Punch

1 (2–ounce) jar instant coffee
1 quart boiling water
2 quarts cold water
1 cup sugar

1 quart chocolate fat–free ice
   cream
1 quart vanilla fat–free ice
   cream

Dissolve coffee and sugar in boiling water. Add cold water. Blend in chocolate ice cream. Chill. For serving, spoon vanilla ice cream into punch bowl and stir gently so that the small scoops of ice cream are floating on top. To serve, scoop vanilla ice cream into punch cups and top with punch.

Fiesta Margaritas

1 (6–ounce) can frozen limeade
   concentrate
6 ounces Triple Sec

6 ounces Cuervo Especial Gold
   tequila
Ice cubes

Pour limeade concentrate into blender. Using limeade can fill with 6 ounces Triple Sec. Pour into blender. Refill limeade can again with 6 ounces tequila and pour into blender. Fill with ice cubes until blender is full. Process until well blended. Pour into margarita glasses and serve at once.

Flavored Iced Tea

1 quart water
2 cups sugar
1 cup lemon juice

1 quart strong tea, steeped and
   cooled
½ teaspoon almond flavoring
1 teaspoon vanilla extract

Boil water; add sugar and stir until dissolves. Add remaining ingredients. Cool. Serve on ice.

Frozen Fruit Slush

2½ cups water
1 cup sugar
1 (6–ounce) can frozen
   lemonade
1 (6–ounce) can frozen orange
   juice

1 (10–ounce) carton frozen
   strawberries
1 (#2) can crushed pineapple
3 bananas, sliced

Boil water and add sugar, stirring until dissolved. Add remaining ingredients. Mix well; freeze. Remove from freezer 30 minutes before serving, while slushy.

Grape Shake

2 cups skim milk
1 cup bottled grape soda

1 pint fat–free vanilla ice cream

Combine milk, soda and half of the ice cream in blender. Process until smooth. To serve, top with remaining ice cream.

Holiday Punch I

1 (6–ounce) can frozen
  lemonade
1 (6–ounce) can frozen orange
  juice concentrate

5 cups water
⅔ cup grenadine syrup
Fresh lemon and orange slices

Combine juices, water and syrup; mix well. Add ginger ale just before serving. Float fruit slices on top.

Holiday Punch II

1 quart cranberry juice, chilled
1 cup sugar
2 cups orange juice, chilled
1 cup pineapple juice, chilled

¾ cup fresh lemon juice,
  chilled
½ teaspoon almond extract
2 cups ginger ale, chilled
1 pint pineapple sherbet

Add first 6 ingredients stirring until sugar is dissolved. Just before serving stir in sherbet. Gently stir in ginger ale.

Hot Fruit Tea

1 teaspoon cinnamon
1 teaspoon cloves
5 teaspoons black tea
24 cups water

Juice of 6 oranges
Juice of 3 lemons
⅛ cup honey
1½ pounds sugar

Tie spices and tea in separate bags. Bring water to a boil. Add tea and spice bags. Heat for 5 minutes. Remove bags. Add fruit juices, honey and sugar. Reheat and serve hot.

Hot Rum Punch

8½ cups apple cider
2 teaspoons pumpkin pie spice
2 to 3 cups light or dark rum to
    taste

12 cinnamon sticks
12 whole cloves

In a large saucepan, bring cider and pumpkin pie spice to a boil. Remove from heat and add rum. Ladle into mugs and add a cinnamon stick and a whole clove to each. Serve at once.

Irish Coffee

2 teaspoons brown sugar
3 tablespoons Irish whiskey
½ cup coffee, freshly brewed

3 tablespoons evaporated
    skimmed milk, chilled and
    whipped

Place sugar and hot coffee in a stemmed glass. Stir to dissolve sugar. Add whiskey. Top with dollop of whipped milk.

Mama's Boiled Custard

3 cups skim milk
⅓ cup sugar
3 Egg Beaters

¼ teaspoon salt
1 teaspoon vanilla extract

Scald milk; let cool down. Add sugar and Egg Beaters. Mix well. Return milk mixture to stove and cook, stirring constantly until mixture coats the spoon. Add salt and vanilla; stir well. Remove from heat and set in pan of cold water until cooled. Refrigerate.

Mocha Au Lait

1 quart skim milk
¼ cup instant chocolate flavor
  mix

2 tablespoons instant coffee
1 tablespoon Cool Whip Lite

Heat milk in heavy saucepan. Add chocolate mix and coffee. Serve piping hot with a dollop of Cool Whip on top.

New Orleans Milk Punch

1½ ounces brandy or bourbon
1½ ounces evaporated
  skimmed milk
1 large scoop fat–free vanilla
  ice cream

¼ teaspoon vanilla extract
⅛ teaspoon nutmeg (optional)
Nutmeg

Mix ingredients in blender. Pour into glass and sprinkle with nutmeg.

October Punch

1 piece of dry ice
2 quarts ginger ale
2 quarts sparkling water
2 (46–ounce) cans pineapple
  juice

1 (6–ounce) can frozen
  lemonade, thawed
1 (6–ounce) can frozen limeade,
  thawed
1 package frozen strawberries

Mix together all ingredients except dry ice. Place dry ice in punch bowl. Pour punch over dry ice.

Orange–Peach Cocktail

1 cup orange juice

¼ cup Peachtree schnapps

Mix together and pour over ice. Makes one serving.

Party Peach Slush

1 (10–ounce) package frozen
  peach slices, partially thawed
1 (6–ounce) can frozen
  lemonade concentrate,
  partially thawed

6 ounces vodka or white rum
1 tablespoon peach schnapps
  liqueur
12 ice cubes

Combine peaches, concentrate, vodka or rum and liqueur. Blend until peaches are chopped. Add ice cubes, one at a time, blending at lowest speed until slushy.

Peach Blossom

2 ounces orange juice
2 ounces peach brandy

4 ounces champagne

Mix well and pour over ice.

Peach Champagne

1 pint fat–free vanilla ice
  cream, softened
2 cups champagne, chilled

1 cup ripe peaches, peeled and
  chopped
Cool Whip Free

Blend ingredients in blender until smooth. Serve at once in stemmed champagne glasses and top with dollop of Cool Whip Free.

Summer Melon Shake

½ cup cantaloupe or honeydew
  melon balls
2 large scoops fat–free vanilla
  ice cream

¼ cup skim milk
1 teaspoon vanilla extract

Place melon balls in blender. Add ice cream, milk, and extract. Process until smooth. Serve immediately.

Pineapple Smoothie

¼ cup pineapple juice
2 tablespoons sugar
1 pint non-fat buttermilk

¼ cup skim milk
3 scoops pineapple sherbet

Place all ingredients in blender and process. Serve icy cold.

Pink "Champagne" Punch

½ cup sugar
1 cup water
1 cup grapefruit juice

½ cup orange juice
¼ cup grenadine syrup
1 large can ginger ale, chilled

Combine sugar and water; simmer until sugar is dissolved. Cool. Add fruit juices and grenadine syrup; chill. Add ginger ale just before serving.

Quick Boiled Custard

1 (5.25-ounce) package French
  vanilla instant pudding
1 cup sugar
1 cup skim milk

1 cup evaporated skimmed
  milk
Vanilla extract to taste

Mix ingredients thoroughly. Chill.

Spiced Tea

½ cup sugar
1½ quarts water
1 cinnamon stick
1 cup instant tea

1 small can orange juice
  concentrate
⅓ cup lemon juice
1 (12-ounce) can pineapple
  juice

Boil sugar, 1 quart water and cinnamon for 5 minutes. Cool. Add remaining ingredients. May be served hot or cold.

Wassail Bowl with Apples

3 large cooking apples, cored
and sliced
1 gallon apple cider
6 whole cloves
6 whole allspice
2 teaspoons nutmeg

1 (6–ounce) can frozen
lemonade concentrate
1 (6–ounce) can frozen orange
juice concentrate
1 cup brown sugar, packed
Cinnamon sticks for garnish

Place sliced apples in a 9 x 13–inch pan and bake at 350° for 25 minutes. Simmer 2 cups apple cider, cloves, allspice and nutmeg for 10 minutes. Add remaining cider, lemonade, juice and brown sugar. Heat until hot but do not boil. Stir occasionally. Pour hot mixture into heated large punch bowl. Float apple, skin sides up, in punch. Sprinkle top of apples with a bit of sugar. To serve, pour hot punch into punch cups. Add cinnamon stick to each serving.

Wintertime Coffee Mix

2 cups fat–free non–dairy
coffee creamer
1½ cups lowfat hot cocoa mix
1½ cups instant coffee

1½ cups sugar
1 teaspoon cinnamon
1 teaspoon ground nutmeg
Pinch of salt

Combine all ingredients, mixing well. Store in a closed container. To serve use 3 tablespoons mix per 1 cup boiling water.

Zippy Tomato Cocktail

2½ cups tomato juice
1 teaspoon onion, grated
½ teaspoon seasoning salt

1½ teaspoons sugar
½ teaspoon Worcestershire
sauce

Combine all ingredients; stir well. Chill for several hours so that flavors can blend.

Condiments

Apple–Cranberry Relish

4 cups cranberries, chopped
1 pound apples
2½ cups brown sugar

1 cup water
½ teaspoon cinnamon

Peel, core and chop apples. Combine all ingredients in large saucepan. Simmer over medium heat for 20 minutes, stirring frequently to prevent sticking. Pour into hot prepared jars, leaving ¼ inch head space. Process 15 minutes in boiling water bath.

Apple–Pumpkin Butter

1 cup canned pumpkin
½ cup applesauce
2 tablespoons honey

¼ teaspoon pumpkin pie spice
Dash salt

Stir all ingredients together in a microwavable container. Cover with plastic wrap leaving one corner open for a vent. Microwave on high 3 to 5 minutes or until thick. Cool to room temperature. Cover and store in refrigerator.

Apricot Spread

1½ quarts apricot pulp
3 cups sugar

2 tablespoons lemon juice

Cook pitted apricots until soft adding enough water to prevent sticking. Press through sieve. Add sugar, cooking over medium heat until thick. Add lemon juice. Pour into hot prepared jars, leaving ¼ inch head space. Adjust caps. Process 10 minutes in boiling water bath.

Aunt Jane's Cranberry Relish

1 package fresh cranberries	2 oranges
1 tart apple, peeled and cored	2 cups sugar
1 lemon	

Grind cranberries in blender. Chop remaining fruits; add sugar. Refrigerate for several hours before serving to allow flavors to blend.

Autumn Chutney

1 pound fresh cranberries	½ teaspoon cloves
1 cup sugar	¼ teaspoon allspice
½ cup brown sugar	1 cup water
½ cup golden raisins	1 cup apple, chopped
2 teaspoons cinnamon	½ cup celery, chopped
1½ teaspoons ginger	½ tablespoon lemon juice

Simmer cranberries, sugars, spices and water in saucepan over medium heat, stirring frequently for 15 minutes. Reduce heat. Add apple, celery and lemon juice. Simmer, uncovered until thick, about 15 minutes. Serve with meats or over fat–free cream cheese as an hors d'oeuvre.

Autumn Pickles

1 gallon whole sour pickles	1 (2½–ounce) box mustard seed
5 pounds sugar	8 cloves garlic, peeled
1 (2–ounce) box peppercorns	

Drain pickles then slice about ¼–inch thick. In the gallon jar, layer pickles, sugar, peppercorns, mustard seed and garlic until all is used. Put lid on. Turn jar over each day until all sugar has dissolved. Let sit in jar for 1 to 2 weeks before serving.

Black Bean Salsa

2 papayas, peeled and cubed
¼ cup fresh pineapple, peeled,
  cored and cubed
½ jalapeño pepper, stemmed,
  seeded and minced

1 teaspoon brown sugar
1 tablespoon fresh lime juice
1 (15–ounce) can black beans,
  rinsed and drained
2 tablespoons fresh cilantro

Mix together well and refrigerate overnight to allow flavors to blend.
Serve with turkey, chicken or pork.

Brandied Blueberry Syrup

7 cups blueberries
9 cups sugar
4 sticks cinnamon, broken in
  half

3 tablespoons lemon juice
¼ cup slivered lemon peel
Dash salt
¼ cup brandy

Mix sugar and blueberries and allow to set 10 hours. Add cinnamon,
lemon juice and peel to berries and place on medium–high heat.
Cook for 20 minutes, stirring frequently so fruit won't stick. Skim
foam from top. Syrup should be thick. Remove from heat and cool.
Add brandy. Stir and seal in prepared jars with paraffin.

Butter Buds Liquid

1 envelope Butter Buds   ½ cup hot tap water

Mix and stir vigorously until fully dissolved. Keep refrigerated.

Christmas Scent

3 (4–inch) sticks cinnamon
3 bay leaves
¼ cup whole cloves

½ lemon, halved
½ orange, halved
1 quart water

Combine all ingredients in a teakettle or saucepan; bring to boil. Reduce heat and slowly simmer as long as desired. Add water, if needed. May be stored in refrigerator several days and reused.

Cissy's Strawberry Preserves

4 cups strawberries, capped
   and washed

3 cups sugar

Pour sugar over berries, stir. Let stand for 1 hour. Cook fast over moderate–high heat for 25 minutes, stirring to prevent sticking. Remove from heat. Let stand until cooled. Pour into hot, sterilized jars and seal.

Citrus Marmalade

3 lemons, thinly sliced
3 limes, thinly sliced

7 cups water
6 to 7 cups sugar

Place lemons and limes in a stainless steel pot. Add water and let stand 24 hours. Bring to a rapid boil and boil over medium heat for 25 minutes. Measure contents and add equal amount of sugar. Return to heat and boil 30 to 40 minutes or until lemon slices are clear and liquid is thick. Pour into prepared jars and seal.

Cranberry Conserve

2 cups water
2 cups brown sugar
6 cups fresh cranberries,
  washed

2 tablespoons orange peel,
  grated
4 oranges, chopped
2 apples, chopped

Mix water and brown sugar in heavy pan. Heat to boil and boil for 2 minutes. Add remaining ingredients. Bring to boil again and cook until cranberries begin to pop.

Cranberry–Raisin Relish

2 cups golden raisins
2 cups orange juice
1 cup water
3 tablespoons fresh lemon
  juice

½ cup sugar
3 cups cranberries, fresh or
  frozen
Pinch of salt

In a 3–quart saucepan, combine raisins, orange juice, water, lemon juice and sugar; bring to a boil over high heat, stirring to dissolve sugar. Reduce heat and simmer for 10 minutes. Add cranberries and salt; simmer an additional 10 minutes or until liquid barely covers solid ingredients. Cool and refrigerate.

Cranberry Relish

2 cups cranberries
½ cup orange juice
1½ cups sugar

1 teaspoon orange rind, grated
1 tablespoon lemon juice

Wash and pick cranberries. Add lemon and orange juice to berries and cook over low heat until skins pop. Rub berries through rough sieve. Add sugar and boil slowly 10 minutes. Add remaining ingredients during last 5 minutes.

Cream Cheese Butter

4 ounces fat–free cream cheese	¼ to ½ teaspoon white pepper
⅛ cup Ultra Promise 70% Less Fat	¾ teaspoon garlic powder
	1½ teaspoons dried chives
⅛ cup Ultra Promise Fat Free	Salt to taste

Mix together all ingredients well. Refrigerate several hours to allow flavors to blend. Delicious spread on sliced Italian or French bread loaves before heating.

Cream Cheese Spread

½ cup fat–free cream cheese

GARLIC AND CHIVES: Add ¼ cup Ultra Promise 70% Fat Free, ½ teaspoon white pepper, ½ teaspoon garlic powder, ½ teaspoon dried chives, and dash of salt.

ORANGE: Add 4 teaspoons confectioners sugar, ½ teaspoon orange extract; stir well.

ALMOND: Add 4 teaspoons confectioners sugar, ½ teaspoon almond extract; stir well.

VANILLA, NUT: Add 4 teaspoons confectioners sugar, ½ teaspoon vanilla, butter and nut flavoring; stir well.

Cucumber–Pineapple Salsa

1 teaspoon sugar	4 ounces seedless cucumber, diced
1 teaspoon cider vinegar	
½ fresh pineapple, peeled, cored and diced	1 shallot, peeled and minced

Mix all ingredients. Refrigerate overnight to allow flavors to blend. May be served with grilled or broiled swordfish, tuna or chicken.

Curried Mayonnaise

¼ teaspoon garlic powder
1 cup Weight Watcher's Fat
  Free Whipped Dressing
¼ teaspoon curry powder
  or to taste

¼ teaspoon coriander powder
  or to taste
½ teaspoon parsley flakes

Mix all ingredients well. Serve with cold cooked chicken or fish.

Dorothy's Cucumbers

1 tablespoon salt
½ cup sugar
¾ cup cider vinegar

2 medium cucumbers, sliced
  paper thin

Place first 3 ingredients in a quart jar. Let set 1 hour. Mix well. Add sliced cucumbers. Refrigerate. Tastes better with age.

Dorothy's Pickled Beets

1 cup brown sugar
1 cup cider vinegar
½ teaspoon minced garlic
½ teaspoon dry mustard
⅛ teaspoon powdered cloves

¼ teaspoon salt
⅛ cup water
1 (#2) can sliced beets
½ small onion, sliced

Put first 7 ingredients in a small saucepan, bring to a boil. Reduce heat and simmer 5 to 7 minutes. Place beets and onion in a container. Pour liquid over all. Let cool then refrigerate.

Easy Vegetable Relish

6 onions
6 green peppers
6 red peppers
1 head cabbage
1 hot pepper

4 cups sugar
1 quart apple cider vinegar
1 tablespoon mustard seed
1 tablespoon celery seed
Salt

Grind vegetables fine. Salt lightly and let stand overnight. Drain and add sugar, vinegar, mustard seed and celery seed. Put in sterilized jars cold. Wait at least 2 weeks before serving.

Ellen's Colonial Mustard

½ cup light brown sugar
⅓ cup prepared mustard
2 Egg Beaters

2 tablespoons Ultra Promise
    70% Fat Free
⅓ cup vinegar

Combine all ingredients in a saucepan. Heat to boiling on medium heat, whisking continually. Cook for 3 minutes.

Fancy Salsa

1 jar mild to medium Old El
    Paso salsa
1½ cups celery, finely chopped
1 cup onion, finely chopped

1 tablespoon dried cilantro
1 can chopped green chilies
    (optional)

Combine all ingredients. Chill. Serve with lowfat chips or on tortillas.

Freezer Apple Pie Filling

6 pounds apples
Fruit fresh
2 cups sugar
¼ cup flour

1½ teaspoons cinnamon
¼ teaspoon nutmeg
¼ teaspoon cloves
2 tablespoons lemon juice

Peel, core and slice apples. Place sliced apples in fruit fresh solution. Combine sugar, flour and spices. Place drained apples into sugar mixture. Let stand 30 minutes. Stir in lemon juice. Cook over medium heat until mixture begins to thicken. Pour into freezer containers and freeze.

Freezer Blueberry Pie Filling

12 cups blueberries
3 cups sugar

¾ cup cornstarch
¼ cup lemon juice

Combine sugar and cornstarch. Add blueberries; let stand for about 30 minutes. Add lemon juice. Cook over medium heat until mixture begin to thicken. May be poured into freezer containers and frozen.

Frosted Grapes

Egg whites
Granulated sugar

Grapes

Beat egg whites until stiff. Dip small bunches of grapes into the egg whites. Let grapes stand until nearly dry on wax paper. Sprinkle with sugar. Let dry thoroughly. May be used as a dessert or a garnish.

Frozen Berries

Raspberries, blueberries,
  blackberries or strawberries
Waxed paper

Baking sheets
Plastic freezer bags

Place fresh berries on waxed papered baking sheet, making sure berries are not touching. Put in freezer until hardened. Remove from freezer and immediately put frozen berries into plastic bags. Seal and return to freezer until ready to use.

Frozen Vegetables

Green peppers, red peppers,
  yellow peppers, onions
  and/or celery

Waxed paper
Baking sheets
Plastic freezer bags

Dice vegetables as you would for cooking. Place vegetables on waxed papered baking sheet, making sure vegetables are not touching. Freeze until hardened. Remove from freezer and immediately put vegetables into plastic bags. Seal and return to freezer until ready to use.

Garden Salsa

¼ pound cucumbers, quartered
1¼ cups red peppers, chopped
⅓ cup red onion, chopped
6 ounces ripe cherry tomatoes,
  peeled

1 large clove garlic, peeled
1½ teaspoons Worcestershire
  sauce
2 tablespoons red wine vinegar

Process vegetables in a food processor until finely chopped. Place in bowl and add remaining ingredients. Refrigerate overnight to allow flavors to blend. May be served with salmon.

Grandmother's Mustard Pickle

1 quart cabbage, chopped
1 quart celery, chopped
1 quart green tomatoes,
    chopped
1 pint green peppers, chopped
1 pint white onions, chopped
1 cup flour, sifted

2 cups sugar
6 tablespoons dry mustard
1 tablespoon turmeric
1 tablespoon celery seed
1 tablespoon mustard seed
3 pints vinegar

Combine first 5 ingredients in a large bowl. Sprinkle with salt and let stand for 1 hour; drain. Meanwhile, mix dry ingredients of remaining ingredients. Add vinegar gradually, stirring constantly. Bring to a boil; add drained vegetables and cook 5 minutes, stirring slowly. Put in prepared pint jars and seal. Makes 8 pints.

Herb Butters

1 tub Ultra Promise Fat Free

ROSEMARY–GARLIC: Add 1½ teaspoons fresh rosemary, finely chopped and ¼ teaspoon garlic.

ITALIAN: Add 1 teaspoon Italian seasonings and 2 tablespoons fat–free Parmesan cheese.

LEMON–THYME: Add 2 teaspoons lemon juice and 1½ teaspoons fresh thyme or 1 teaspoon ground thyme.

GARLIC: Add 1 teaspoon garlic powder.

HONEY: Add 3 tablespoons honey.

First 4 herb butters are delicious spread on sliced Italian or French bread loaves before heating.

Herbed Cream Cheese Spread

½ tablespoon fat–free sour
   cream
½ tablespoon fat–free cream
   cheese
½ tablespoon honey mustard

1 tablespoon fresh basil,
   chopped
½ tablespoon flat leaf parsley,
   chopped

Mix sour cream and cream cheese thoroughly. Add remaining ingredients; stir well. Keep refrigerated.

Holiday Pickles

1 gallon sour pickles
Sugar
Cinnamon sticks

Fresh garlic pods
Maraschino cherries

Drain pickles and cut into large chunks. For a 1–pint jar, layer pickles, 2 to 3 garlic pods and 6 to 8 cherries to fill line. Push 2 cinnamon sticks down sides of jar. Pour 1 cup sugar on top of all. Seal and let sit for 1 weeks. Turn upside down for 1 week, then return to upright position for 1 week. They will be ready to eat in three weeks.

Homemade Hot Dog Relish

5 cups cucumbers, ground
3 cups onions, ground
3 cups celery, finely chopped
2 red peppers, ground
2 green peppers, ground
¾ cup salt

1½ quarts water
1 quart white vinegar
3 cups sugar
2 teaspoons mustard seed
2 teaspoons celery seed

Combine first 7 ingredients and let set overnight; drain. In a Dutch oven heat the remaining ingredients and bring to a boil. Add vegetable mixture and cook 10 minutes. Seal in prepared jars.

Horseradish Mayonnaise

4 tablespoons Reese prepared
  horseradish or to taste

1 cup Weight Watcher's Fat
  Free Whipped Dressing
½ teaspoon parsley

Stir ingredients together. Serve with hot or cold roast beef sandwiches, tenderloin and poached or smoked fish.

Lemon Marmalade

6 lemons, thinly sliced
7 cups water

6 to 7 cups sugar

Place lemons in stainless steel pot and cover with water. Let stand 24
hours. Bring to a rapid boil and boil over medium heat for 25
minutes. Measure contents and add equal amount of sugar. Return
to heat and boil 30 to 40 minutes or until lemons are clear and liquid
is thick. Pour into prepared jars and seal.

Late Summer Relish

4 pounds pears, peeled and
  cored
6 green peppers
6 red peppers
6 onions

1 tablespoon celery seed
1 tablespoon salt
3 cups sugar
1 tablespoon allspice

Grind pears, peppers and onions in food chopped or processor. Add
all ingredients together and boil 30 minutes. Put in prepared jars and
seal.

Marinated Cauliflower

2 large cauliflower, cut in
flowerets
1½ cups peeled tiny onions
¼ cup salt
4 cups white vinegar

2 cups sugar
2 tablespoons mustard seed
1 tablespoon celery seed
1 teaspoon turmeric

Cover prepared cauliflowerets, salt and onions with ice. Let stand 3 hours. Drain thoroughly. Bring next 5 ingredients to a boil. Add vegetables and return to a boil. Reduce heat and simmer 7 minutes. Pack into hot, prepared jars, leaving ¼ inch head space. Adjust caps. Process 10 minutes in boiling water bath.

Marinated Onions

3 large onions, thinly sliced
3 tablespoons Tabasco

3 tablespoons red wine vinegar

Pour boiling water over onions and let stand 1 minute; drain. Mix Tabasco and vinegar. Pour over onion rings. Refrigerate for at least 3 hours before serving. May be drained before serving.

Mixed Fruit Jam

3 pounds ripe peaches (4 cups
mashed)
3 pounds sugar (6¾ cups)

2 oranges
1 small jar maraschino cherries,
chopped

Combine sugar and peaches and let set overnight. Next morning add juice and pulp of oranges plus grated orange rind of 1 orange and cherries with juice. Cook together for 1 hour. Pour into prepared jars and seal.

Muscadine Syrup

2½ pounds muscadines
1¾ cups sugar

⅓ cup corn syrup
1 tablespoon lemon juice

Wash and crush muscadines. Cook over low heat 10 to 20 minutes. Put through a food mill or sieve; discard hulls and seeds. Measure 1½ cups puree in a saucepan; add sugar, corn syrup and lemon juice. Bring to a full boil and boil 2 minutes. Remove from heat, remove foam; pour into container. Makes about 3 cups. May be canned by pouring into prepared jars, leaving ¼ inch head space. Adjust lids. Process in boiling water bath, 212°, for 10 minutes.

Orange Marmalade

1 lemon
3 oranges
3 cups water

2 cups sugar
Scant pinch of salt

1ST DAY: Grind fruit. Add water and let set mixture aside overnight.

2ND DAY: Bring to a boil and cook 10 minutes. Set aside overnight.

3RD DAY: Gradually add sugar and salt. Cook to jelly stage. Pour into prepared jars and seal.

Peach Salsa

1 teaspoon brown sugar
1 tablespoon fresh lime juice
1 tablespoon fresh ginger, grated
2 tablespoons cilantro, chopped

4 large ripe peaches, peeled, seeded and chopped
Pinch of salt
Fresh lime zest, grated

Add all ingredients. Refrigerate overnight to allow flavors to blend.

Pineapple–Pear Honey

8 cups ripe pears
2 cups crushed pineapple

4 cups sugar
Juice of 1 lemon

Wash, pare and core pears. Slice before measuring out 8 cups. Put pears through food grinder or finely chop. Combine pears, pineapple, sugar and lemon juice. Cook 20 to 30 minutes stirring frequently. Pour into prepared jars and seal.

Pineapple–Rum Syrup

2 fresh pineapples, peeled,
  cored and cut into chunks
2 cups water

2 cinnamon sticks, broken
1½ cups brown sugar
½ cup rum

Combine water, brown sugar and cinnamon sticks; bring to a boil; reduce heat and simmer 5 minutes, stirring occasionally. Add pineapple; simmer in syrup until heated through. Remove from heat; stir in rum. Pack into hot, prepared jars leaving ¼ inch head space. Adjust caps. Process 15 minutes in boiling water bath.

Pineapple–Mango Salsa

½ large pineapple, peeled,
  cored and diced
1 ripe mango, peeled, pitted
  and diced
½ jalapeño pepper, stemmed,
  seeded and minced

2 tablespoons red onion, finely
  chopped
1 tablespoon fresh lime juice
2 tablespoons cilantro,
  chopped
Pinch of salt

In a bowl combine pineapple and mango; toss. Add remaining ingredients. Stir well. Refrigerate overnight to allow flavors to blend. May be served with crab.

Raspberry Freezer Jam

1 quart fresh raspberries
4 cups sugar
1 tablespoon framboise
   (raspberry liqueur)

1 cup water
2 tablespoons powdered pectin
1 teaspoon lemon juice

In a large bowl, mash berries. Add sugar and liqueur; let stand 10 minutes. Strain through a fine sieve. In a small saucepan, mix water, pectin and lemon juice and bring to a boil for 1 minute, stirring constantly. Remove from heat, add to puree and stir well. Ladle into freezer container. Refrigerate until thoroughly cooled and freeze.

Red and Green Pepper Relish

7 cups red peppers, finely
   chopped
3 cups green peppers, finely
   chopped

4 cups onions, finely chopped
3 tablespoons salt
2 cups sugar
2 cups cider vinegar

Combine all ingredients in kettle. Bring to a boil and simmer 1 hour. Pour at once into hot, sterile jars. Seal.

Simmering Christmas Potpourri

½ orange peel
¼ cup cloves
1 cinnamon stick

½ lemon peel
2 bay leaves

Simmer in uncovered pot for a lovely aroma.

Simmering Holiday Potpourri

1 grapefruit peel
2 lemon peels
1 tablespoon cloves

2 orange peels
2 cinnamon sticks
1 teaspoon allspice

Mix together in simmering pot for a festive scent.

Spiced Apple Butter

9 to 10 Rome apples, washed and diced
9 to 10 Granny Smith apples, washed and diced
1 cup water

4 cups sugar
1½ teaspoons cinnamon
½ teaspoon cloves
2 tablespoons fresh lemon juice

Combine apples and water and cook until done. Press through a food mill. This should measure 12 cups. Return to saucepan. Heat 2 cups of sugar in a saucepan, stirring until sugar melts and turns a golden brown. Carefully pour into apple pulp. Sugar will crackle and harden. Add remaining sugar and spices. Cook, uncovered for 1 hour, stirring occasionally to prevent sticking. Stir in lemon juice. Pour into prepared jars leaving ¼ inch head space. Adjust caps. Process 10 minutes in a boiling water bath.

Spicy Red Tomato Relish

2 quarts ripe tomatoes, peeled and quartered
½ cup vinegar
1 teaspoon salt

1 cup sugar
1 cup onion, chopped
½ cup green pepper, chopped
2 to 3 hot peppers, chopped

Mix together all ingredients. Cook over low heat for approximately 2 hours. Seal in prepared jars.

Tomato Relish Spread

4½ pounds ripe tomatoes, peeled and seeded
1½ pounds sugar
¼ teaspoon cloves

¼ teaspoon cinnamon
¼ teaspoon allspice
1 cup vinegar

Combine all ingredients and cook for about 1½ hours or until mixture becomes very thick. Cook over low heat and stir often. When mixture reaches a spreadable consistency, bring to a boil and pack into sterile jars. Seal. Process in water bath at 212° for 20 minutes.

Creamy Tarragon Dressing

1 cup non–fat buttermilk
½ cup Weight Watcher's Fat
  Free Whipped Dressing

2 teaspoons tarragon

Mix all ingredients well. Refrigerate for several hours allowing flavors to blend. May be served cold or heated before serving.

Dijon Basil Vinaigrette

1 cup fat–free Italian dressing
1 teaspoon sugar

2 teaspoons Dijon mustard
1 teaspoon dried basil

Mix together all ingredients. Keep refrigerated.

Dijon Tarragon Vinaigrette

1 cup fat–free Italian dressing
1 teaspoon sugar

2 teaspoons Dijon mustard
1 teaspoon dried tarragon

Mix together all ingredients. Keep refrigerated.

Honey–Mustard Dressing

½ cup Weight Watcher's Fat
  Free Whipped Dressing
¼ cup honey
¼ cup mustard

¼ cup skim milk
½ to ¾ teaspoon black pepper
  or to taste

Mix all ingredients well. Keep refrigerated.

Lime Dressing

1 cup fat–free ranch dressing
4 teaspoons fresh lime peel,
  grated
1 tablespoon fresh lime juice

1 teaspoon sugar
¼ teaspoon ground round
  pepper

Combine all ingredients stirring until sugar dissolves. Keep refrigerated.

Orange Vinaigrette

½ cup fat–free Italian dressing
¼ cup sugar

¼ cup orange juice

Combine all ingredients and stir until sugar dissolves.

Poppy Seed Dressing

1 cup fat–free Italian dressing
½ cup sugar

4 teaspoons poppy seed

Mix together dressing and sugar; stir until sugar dissolves. Add poppy seeds.

Raspberry Vinaigrette

½ cup fat–free Italian dressing
¼ cup sugar

¼ cup frozen raspberries

Combine all ingredients in a blender. Process until smooth.

Roquefort Cream Dressing

1 cup Kraft Free blue cheese
1 tablespoon fat–free sour
  cream

¼ teaspoon garlic powder
⅛ teaspoon onion powder
1 teaspoon dried parsley

Mix all ingredients together. Refrigerate.

NOTE: For thinner consistency, add skim milk as desired.

Sweet and Sour Dressing

1 cup fat–free Italian dressing   ½ cup sugar

Mix together. Stir until sugar dissolves.

Vinaigrette Dressing

¼ cup fat–free Italian dressing   1 cup skim milk
⅜ cup Dijon mustard

Combine all ingredients and mix well. More milk may be added if a thinner consistency is desired.

VARIATIONS: Tarragon: Add 1½ teaspoons dried tarragon to ingredients.

Italian: Add 1½ teaspoons dried Italian seasonings to ingredients.

Basil: Add 1½ teaspoons dried basil to ingredients.

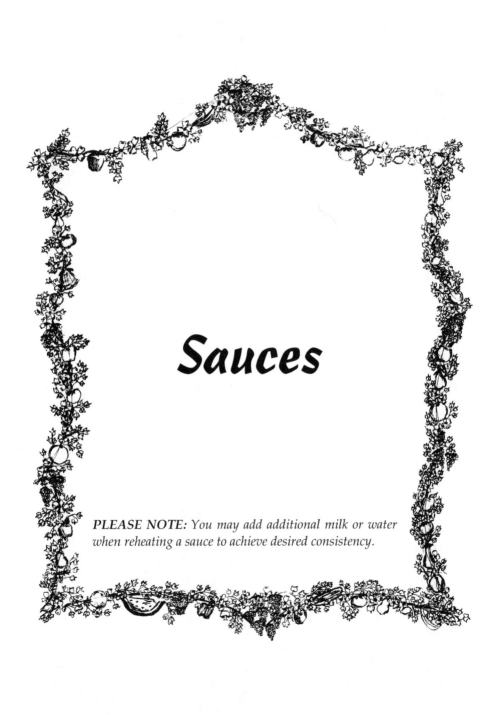

Sauces

PLEASE NOTE: *You may add additional milk or water when reheating a sauce to achieve desired consistency.*

Heavenly Sauce

1 cup sugar
½ cup non–fat buttermilk
2 tablespoons Ultra Promise
  70% Less Fat
6 tablespoons Fleischmann's
  Fat Free Squeezable Spread

½ teaspoon soda
½ teaspoon butter extract
1 teaspoon vanilla extract
1 tablespoon white corn syrup

Combine all ingredients in a saucepan and bring to a boil stirring constantly. Serve hot over slices of angel food cake.

Apricot Sauce

1 cup dried apricots
1 cup water
½ cup sugar

1 (8–ounce) can crushed
  pineapple

Place apricots and water in heavy saucepan and cook, covered, over very low heat until fruit falls apart when stirred. Add sugar and stir until dissolved. Add pineapple with juice. Bring mixture to a boil. Remove from heat. Serve warm.

Banana Sauce

¾ cup sugar
¼ cup + ⅛ cup skim milk
⅛ cup Butter Buds Liquid
  (see page 50)
½ teaspoon Ultra Promise 70%
  Less Fat

½ teaspoon vanilla extract
½ tablespoon flour
1 small banana
Lemon juice

Mash banana and squeeze a small amount of lemon juice on banana; set aside. In a medium saucepan add remaining ingredients. Cook until spoon is coated; add banana. Serve warm if desired.

Barbecue Sauce

1 cup ketchup
½ cup distilled vinegar
½ cup Worcestershire sauce
1 package Butter Buds Powder
1 teaspoon mustard

2 tablespoons sugar
1 teaspoon salt
1 cup onion, finely chopped
3 tablespoons brown sugar

Sauté onions in a non–stick Pam–sprayed skillet. Combine all ingredients. Simmer for 15 minutes. May be served hot or cold.

Blackberry Sauce

1½ cups sugar
⅓ cup cornstarch
4 cups fresh or frozen
   blackberries

1½ tablespoons Fleischmann's
   Fat Free Squeezable Spread
1 tablespoon fresh lemon juice
1 cup water
1 teaspoon lemon rind, grated

Combine all ingredients and cook over low heat. Stir with whisk until smooth. Serve warm or cold.

Bourbon Sauce

3 tablespoons Ultra Promise
   70% Less Fat
1 tablespoon Fleischmann's Fat
   Free Squeezable Spread
1 cup sugar

1 Egg Beater
¼ cup skim (or evaporated
   skimmed) milk
¼ cup bourbon

In top of double boiler melt Promise, Fleischmann's and sugar. Gradually whisk in Egg Beater, then milk. Heat until hot and thick. Cool slightly and add bourbon. Serve warm.

Brandy Sauce

¾ cup Egg Beater
9 tablespoons sugar
3 tablespoons brandy

¾ cup evaporated skimmed
   milk

Combine Egg Beaters, sugar and milk in top of double boiler. Beat vigorously with whisk. Place pan over (not in) simmering water. Beat for 10 minutes or until mixture is thick. Remove from heat and add brandy.

Cheese Sauce

1½ tablespoons Fleischmann's
   Fat Free Squeezable Spread
1½ tablespoons flour
½ cup chicken bouillon
1 cup evaporated skimmed
   milk
¼ teaspoon salt

¼ teaspoon white pepper
1 ounce (¼ cup) Kroger Lite
   Classics Sharp Cheddar
   longhorn style cheese,
   shredded
¾ cup fat–free Cheddar cheese,
   shredded

Blend Fleischmann's and flour in saucepan. Gradually whisk bouillon and milk into flour mixture. Cook on medium heat, stirring constantly until thick. Add salt and pepper. Add cheeses. Heat until cheese melts.

Cocktail Sauce

¾ cup chili sauce
4 tablespoons fresh lemon
   juice or to taste

2 teaspoons Worcestershire
   sauce
½ teaspoon onions, grated
4 drops Tabasco sauce

Combine all ingredients and chill for several hours before serving.

Cranberry Glaze

1 (16–ounce) can whole
  cranberry sauce
½ cup Burgundy
6 whole cloves

1 cup brown sugar
2½ teaspoons prepared
  mustard
1 teaspoon lemon juice

Mix all ingredients together in a saucepan. Simmer uncovered for 5 minutes.

May be used as a glaze for ham.

Cranberry and Horseradish Sauce

1 (1–pound) can whole berry
  cranberry sauce
1 tablespoon Reese prepared
  horseradish

1 teaspoon fresh orange rind,
  grated

Mix together. Serve with cold turkey, chicken or pork.

Cranberry–Orange Sauce

1 (14–ounce) can whole
  cranberry sauce

1 (8–ounce) jar orange
  marmalade

In a small mixing bowl, combine cranberry sauce and marmalade until well blended. Cover and chill in the refrigerator before serving.

Dijon Sauce

3 tablespoons Dijon mustard
2 tablespoons fat–free Italian
  salad dressing

1 teaspoon Weight Watcher's
  Fat Free Whipped Dressing
¼ teaspoon black pepper

Combine all ingredients and mix well.

73

Easy Brown Sauce

1½ tablespoons Ultra Promise
   70% Less Fat
1½ tablespoons Fleischmann's
   Fat Free Squeezable Spread
3 tablespoons flour

1½ cups beef broth
½ teaspoon thyme
Salt to taste
Pepper to taste

Make a paste with Promise, Fleischmann's and flour. Add beef broth and thyme. Whisk briskly to remove lumps. Heat, whisking until sauce thickens. Add salt and pepper. Reduce heat and simmer until warmed thoroughly.

Fruit Salad Dressing

½ cup sugar
1 teaspoon salt
3 tablespoons flour
¼ teaspoon powdered ginger
2 Egg Beaters

¼ cup vinegar
1 cup pineapple juice
½ cup orange juice
1 teaspoon orange rind, grated

Place all dry ingredients in saucepan. Add Egg Beaters and mix thoroughly. Add vinegar, juices and orange rind. Cook over low heat until thick and smooth, stirring constantly. Chill.

Genuine Teriyaki Sauce

1 cup soy sauce
¾ cup water
1½ tablespoons bourbon
2 tablespoons sugar

1 tablespoon confectioners
   sugar
½ teaspoon garlic powder

Combine all ingredients. Marinate beef or chicken 12 to 24 hours before cooking or barbecuing.

Grand Mariner Sauce

¾ cup Egg Beaters
9 tablespoons sugar
3 tablespoons Grand Marnier

¾ cup evaporated skimmed
 milk

Combine Egg Beaters, sugar and milk in top of double boiler. Beat with whisk or electric beater. Place pan over (not in) simmering water. Beat for about 10 minutes or until mixture is thick. Remove from heat. Add Grand Marnier; stir.

Italian Vinaigrette Dressing

½ cup red wine vinegar
2 teaspoons Dijon mustard
1 teaspoon sugar

1½ cups fat–free Italian
 dressing
Salt and pepper to taste

Mix all ingredients together, using a whisk. Keep refrigerated.

Linda's Ginger–Apricot Sauce

½ cup sugar
2 tablespoons cornstarch
⅛ teaspoon ginger
1 tablespoon fresh lemon juice

½ teaspoon lemon rind, freshly
 grated
1 cup pineapple juice
1 (12–ounce) can apricot nectar

Mix together sugar, cornstarch, ginger and lemon rind. Stir in juices until smooth. Cook over medium heat; bring to a boil and simmer for 10 minutes, stirring constantly. Remove from heat; let cool, stirring occasionally.

Madeira Sauce

1 recipe Quick Brown Sauce
 (see page 75)

½ cup Madeira wine

Mix together and simmer until heated thoroughly.

Lemon Sauce I

1 tablespoon Ultra Promise
   70% Less Fat
1 tablespoon flour
1½ tablespoons fresh lemon
   juice

½ cup boiling water
¼ cup sugar
1 teaspoon lemon rind, grated
1 drop yellow food coloring

Make a paste with Promise and flour. Whisk lemon juice and water into flour mixture, briskly. Add sugar, rind and coloring. Cook over low heat, stirring constantly until slightly thickened. Serve warm.

Lemon Sauce II

2 tablespoons flour
1 tablespoon Ultra Promise
   70% Less Fat
1 tablespoon Fleischmann's Fat
   Free Squeezable Spread
1½ cups water

3 tablespoons fresh lemon
   juice
1 cup sugar
2 Egg Beaters
Lemon peel, grated

Make a paste with flour, Promise and Fleischmann's. Add water and lemon juice; whisking well. On low heat, whisk mixture until all lumps are gone. Add sugar, Egg Beaters and lemon peel. Stir until thick.

Mustard Sauce

½ cup brown sugar
½ cup vinegar
2 tablespoons dry mustard
2 tablespoons Ultra Promise
   70% Less Fat

2 tablespoons Fleischmann's
   Fat Free Squeezable Spread
2 Egg Beaters
Dash of salt

Put all ingredients in top of double boiler and stir over medium heat until thickened. Serve with fat–free cocktail sausages, seafood, ham or beef.

No–Cook Caramel Sauce

¾ cup brown sugar
1 tablespoon Ultra Promise
  70% Less Fat
1 tablespoon Fleischmann's Fat
  Free Squeezable Spread

¼ teaspoon salt
½ cup hot evaporated skimmed
  milk

Put all ingredients into blender. Cover and process on mix until sugar is dissolved.

Onion Sauce

2 medium to large onions
2 cups skim milk
½ teaspoon nutmeg
Salt and pepper to taste
1 bay leaf

2 tablespoons Ultra Promise
  70% Less Fat
2 tablespoons Fleischmann's
  Fat Free Squeezable Spread
½ cup flour

Cut onions into eighths. In a heavy saucepan, cook onions in milk with nutmeg, salt and pepper and bay leaf. Cook until onions are soft. Remove bay leaf. Strain this mixture and reserve liquid and onions separately. Make a paste with Promise, Fleischmann's and flour. Add this to the milk mixture. Whisk briskly until all the lumps are gone. Heat slowly. If desired, add onions and heat through. Serve hot with steaks, rabbit, and boiled lamb.

Pizza Sauce

1 (24–ounce) can tomato puree
½ cup stewed tomatoes
4 teaspoons sugar
1½ teaspoons salt
½ tablespoon sherry

1½ teaspoons garlic, crushed
½ teaspoon oregano
¼ teaspoon basil
¼ teaspoon marjoram
1 teaspoon Italian seasoning

Combine all ingredients in a medium saucepan. Bring to a slow simmer, stirring occasionally. Must simmer for several hours, until consistency is thick and deep red in color.

Orange Sauce I

½ cup sugar
1 tablespoon cornstarch
1 cup orange juice, boiling
2 tablespoons Ultra Promise
  70% Less Fat

1½ tablespoons lemon juice
Dash of nutmeg
Dash of salt

Mix sugar and cornstarch. Add juice, gradually, stirring constantly. Cover and boil gently until thick, stirring occasionally. Remove from heat. Add remaining ingredients. Makes 1 cup.

Orange Sauce II

¾ cup orange juice

¾ cup sugar

Stir well until sugar is dissolved.

Pepper A La King Sauce

2 tablespoons Ultra Promise
  70% Less Fat
2 tablespoons Fleischmann's
  Fat Free Squeezable Spread
¼ green pepper, cored, seeded
  and cut in short, thin strips
¼ red pepper, cored, seeded
  and cut in short, thin strips

⅓ cup flour
Salt to taste
¼ teaspoon white pepper
1 cup evaporated skimmed
  milk
1 cup water
2 tablespoons dry sherry

In a non–stick Pam–sprayed skillet, sauté vegetables until tender. In a saucepan, make a paste out of Ultra Promise, Fleischmann's and flour. Add milk and water. Whisk mixture briskly until most of lumps are out. Heat slowly, constantly whisking until smooth. Add sautéed vegetables, salt, pepper and sherry. Heat through. Serve hot with chicken breasts.

Pepper Sherry Sauce

⅛ cup Ultra Promise 70% Less
   Fat
⅛ cup Fleischmann's Fat Free
   Squeezable Spread
1 small carrot, chopped
1 celery rib, chopped
1 bay leaf

1 fresh thyme sprig
2 teaspoons flour
1 cup red wine
1 tablespoon red wine vinegar
¼ teaspoon freshly ground
   pepper

In a non–stick Pam–sprayed skillet, sauté vegetables. Meanwhile, warm wine vinegar, bay leaf and thyme in a saucepan. Let set for 10 minutes. Make a paste out of Promise, Fleischmann's and flour. Add wine mixture that has been strained. Whisk mixture briskly to remove all lumps. Bring to a boil and gently simmer. Add pepper to taste. Cook until desired consistency. Serve hot with beef or venison.

Plantation Sauce

1 (10–ounce) jar apple jelly
1 (10–ounce) jar pineapple
   preserves
1 (5–ounce) jar Reese
   horseradish

1 (5–ounce) jar mustard
1 teaspoon sugar
1 teaspoon lemon juice

In saucepan melt jelly. Add remaining ingredients. Keep refrigerated. Serve with ham.

Quick Horseradish Sauce

1 cup Weight Watcher's Fat
   Free Whipped Dressing
½ cup Reese horseradish

½ teaspoon prepared mustard
¼ teaspoon ground mustard

Mix all ingredients well. Serve with beef tenderloin or steak.

Prune Sauce

1 (7–ounce) package pitted
  prunes
2 tablespoons fresh lemon
  juice
1 tablespoon lemon peel, finely
  grated
8 whole cloves

Ground cinnamon
Ground allspice
½ teaspoon nutmeg
½ cup sugar
1 tablespoon Fleischmann's Fat
  Free Squeezable Spread
½ cup red wine vinegar

In a saucepan add first 9 ingredients and cook slowly for 15 minutes. Puree in food processor. Return to saucepan. Add wine vinegar. Cook over low heat and stir until smooth and warmed through. Serve with roast pork.

Raisin Sauce

½ cup brown sugar
1 tablespoon mustard
¼ teaspoon ginger
¼ cup distilled vinegar
1¼ cups water
2 cinnamon sticks

2 whole cloves
1 tablespoon cornstarch
1 tablespoon water
½ cup raisins
⅓ cup dry sherry
Salt to taste

In a small saucepan, mix first seven ingredients. Simmer for 10 minutes. Thicken with cornstarch and water. Remove from heat. Add raisins, sherry and salt. Serve warm over turkey ham or pork.

Raspberry–Strawberry Sauce

2 cups fresh strawberries,
  hulled

2 cups raspberries, fresh or
  frozen, thawed
1 cup sugar

Combine fruit in blender and puree. Add sugar.

Rebel Sauce

½ cup Butter Buds Liquid
    (see page 50)
1 cup confectioners sugar

½ cup cold water
1½ teaspoons vanilla extract
1 tablespoon cornstarch

Add all ingredients, except vanilla, in a medium saucepan and cook until spoon is coated. Add vanilla. Serve warm.

Rich Fudge Sauce

1 (12–ounce) can evaporated
    skimmed milk
1¼ cups sugar
¼ cup cocoa

¼ cup Fleischmann's Fat Free
    Squeezable Spread
1 teaspoon vanilla extract
½ teaspoon salt

Mix all ingredients in a medium saucepan. Bring to a boil, stirring frequently. Cook for 2 minutes. Let cool and refrigerate.

Spaghetti Sauce

½ pound ground round
1 cup onion, diced
⅓ cup bell pepper, diced
1 teaspoon minced garlic
1 (14–ounce) can stewed
    tomatoes
1 (12–ounce) can Italian tomato
    paste

1¼ teaspoons salt
1¼ teaspoons garlic salt
½ teaspoon pepper
1 teaspoon basil
1 teaspoon oregano
1 bay leaf
1 tablespoon sugar

In a non–stick Pam–sprayed skillet, sauté onions and bell pepper. Meanwhile cook ground round in a colander in a microwave until done. Add all ingredients in skillet with onions and peppers. Simmer for 1½ hours, stirring occasionally. May be served on spaghetti noodles or in casseroles.

Sherry Wine Sauce

⅓ cup currant jelly
⅓ cup ketchup
⅓ cup sherry

1 teaspoon sugar
Dash of salt

In a saucepan, melt jelly. Add remaining ingredients. Serve warm.

Sun–dried Tomato Spread

7 ounces sun–dried tomatoes
2 (8–ounce) packages fat–free
    cream cheese
4 green onions

12 fresh basil leaves
Dash Worcestershire sauce
1 teaspoon dried chives
Baguette slices

Chop tomatoes in food processor and set aside. Combine cream cheese and next 4 ingredients in food processor and process until smooth. Spread mixture in a circle on a platter. Cover with chopped tomatoes and chill at least 4 hours. Serve with baguette slices.

Summer Ham Sauce

½ cup water
Juice of 2 large lemons
Salt to taste
¼ cup light brown sugar,
    firmly packed
Zest of one lemon, grated

2 tablespoons Ultra Promise
    70% Less Fat
2 tablespoons Fleischmann's
    Fat Free Squeezable Spread
¼ cup flour
⅓ cup seedless raisins

Warm water, lemon juice, salt, brown sugar and lemon rind; set aside. In a saucepan, make a paste out of Promise, Fleischmann's and flour. Add lemon juice mixture and whisk briskly to remove all lumps. Add raisins. Warm slowly until raisins are warmed through. Serve with ham.

Turkey Gravy

2 (14.5–ounce) cans chicken
  broth
4 hard–boiled egg whites,
  finely chopped

½ cup turkey breast, cooked
  and finely diced
Salt and pepper to taste
2 tablespoons cornstarch
2 tablespoons water

Bring chicken broth to a boil. Add egg whites, turkey, salt and pepper. In a separate container, mix together cornstarch and water. Add to broth mixture. Cook over medium heat, stirring constantly, until thickened. Serve hot with Cornbread Dressing.

NOTE: A thicker gravy may be achieved by adding more cornstarch and water, if desired.

Vanilla Sauce

⅓ cup sugar
1 tablespoon cornstarch
Pinch of salt

2 cups skim milk
2 Egg Beaters
2 teaspoons vanilla extract

In a medium saucepan combine sugar, cornstarch and salt. Whisk in milk and Egg Beaters. Bring to a boil over medium–low heat, stirring constantly. Cook and stir for 1 minute after mixture comes to a boil and thickens. Remove from heat; add vanilla. May be served warm over pound cake.

Vegetable Sauce

1 can Campbell's Healthy
  Request cream of mushroom
  soup
1½ tablespoons Ultra Promise
  70% Less Fat

3 tablespoons Fleischmann's
  Fat Free Squeezable Spread
1 cup fat–free Cheddar cheese,
  shredded

In a small saucepan, mix all ingredients, heating just until cheese melts, stirring constantly. Serve over hot vegetables.

White Cocktail Sauce

1 cup Weight Watcher's Fat
  Free Whipped Dressing
1 (5–ounce) jar Kraft's
  horseradish
4 teaspoons onion, grated

1 teaspoon lemon juice
¼ teaspoon garlic powder
Salt to taste
White pepper to taste

Mix all ingredients and refrigerate for several hours before serving.

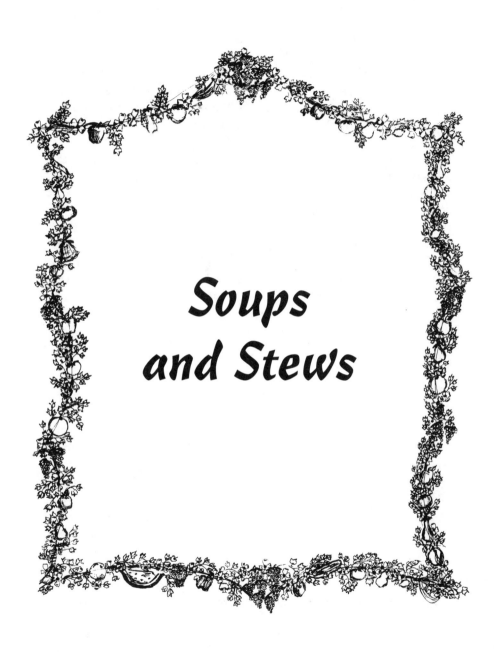

Soups
and Stews

Autumn Stew

2 pounds top round steak, cut
  into bite–sized pieces
4 medium onions, chopped
3 cloves garlic, pressed
2 large green peppers, chopped
2 large tomatoes, peeled and
  chopped
1 tablespoon salt or to taste
1½ teaspoons black pepper
2 tablespoons Fleischmann's
  Fat Free Squeezable Spread

5 cans beef broth
2 dozen dried prunes
6 ounces dried apricots
6 ounces dried apples
6 yams, peeled and cubed
4 (10–ounce) packages whole
  kernel corn
¾ cup red wine
1 pumpkin, 9–quart size

In a Pam–sprayed non–stick skillet sauté meat until done and put in a large kettle. Sauté onions, garlic and green peppers in Pam–sprayed non–stick skillet; add to meat in kettle. Mix remaining ingredients, except for pumpkin. Cook slowly for 1 hour. Cut top off of pumpkin, remove seeds and membrane. Fill pumpkin with stew. Bake at 325° for 1 hour. Place pumpkin on platter and serve from it.

Bean and Bacon Soup

1 pound dried navy beans
7 cups water
1½ teaspoons salt or to taste
¼ teaspoon pepper or to taste
1 teaspoon garlic, minced
1 bay leaf

3 slices Oscar Mayer Bacon
1½ cups onions, finely diced
¾ cup green pepper, finely
  diced
½ cup finely chopped carrots
1 (8–ounce) can tomato sauce

Sort and wash beans; place in Dutch oven. Add water, garlic and bay leaf. Cook 2 hours. Add bacon slices and continue to simmer 45 minutes to 1 hour or until beans are tender. Sauté onions and peppers in a Pam–sprayed non–stick skillet. Add onions, peppers, carrots, salt and pepper to bean mixture. Simmer 30 minutes. Add tomato sauce and simmer an additional 30 minutes. Remove bacon and bay leaf before serving.

Beef Consommé

2 cups Burgundy
4 cups beef consommé
3 cups V–8 juice

1 cup lemon juice
1 tablespoon sugar

Combine; stir until sugar is dissolved. Serve hot or cold.

Broccoli–Cheese Soup

1 (10–ounce) package broccoli, frozen
2 tablespoons onion, finely chopped
½ teaspoon salt
¼ teaspoon pepper
1 cup chicken broth
3 tablespoons Fleischmann's Fat Free Squeezable Spread

3 tablespoons flour
2 cups evaporated skimmed milk
¼ cup Kroger Lite Classics sharp Cheddar cheese, shredded
¾ cup fat–free Cheddar cheese, shredded

Cook broccoli, onion, salt and pepper in chicken broth. Make a paste with Fleischmann's and flour. Using a whisk, gradually add milk to flour mixture. On low heat, cook this mixture, stirring constantly, until it begins to thicken. Add this to the broccoli mixture and continue to cook until thick. Add cheeses and simmer until cheese melts.

NOTE: For thinner soup, substitute ½ of evaporated skimmed milk with regular skim milk.

Cauliflower Soup

1 head cauliflower, chopped
4 green onions, chopped
1 large apple, chopped
5 cups chicken broth

1 cup white wine
1 tablespoon lemon juice
Tabasco sauce to taste
Salt and pepper to taste

Simmer cauliflower, onions and apple in broth for 30 minutes. Strain broth. Puree solids. Return puree to broth and add remaining ingredients. Heat thoroughly but do not boil.

Cajun Jambalaya

2 medium onions, chopped
2 green peppers, chopped
6 green onions, chopped
1 (16–ounce) can stewed
   tomatoes
1 (6–ounce) can tomato paste
1 teaspoon salt
¼ cup Fleischmann's Fat Free
   Squeezable Spread

2½ cups chicken breasts,
   cooked and diced fine
½ pound turkey ham, diced
   fine
½ pound fat–free smoked
   turkey sausage, diced fine
1¾ cups rice, cooked
4 cups water
¾ teaspoon Tabasco

Sauté onions, peppers and green onions in a non–stick Pam–sprayed skillet. In a stew pot, add sautéed vegetables, tomatoes, tomato paste and salt. Simmer, covered, for 10 minutes. Add Fleischmann's, chicken, turkey ham, sausage, rice and water. Bring to a slow simmer, covered, for 1 hour, stirring frequently. Add additional water or chicken broth, if desired. Stir in Tabasco just before serving.

Cabbage Soup

1 (46–ounce) can tomato juice
1½ heads cabbage, shredded
   fine
½ cup green pepper, chopped
   fine
1 tablespoon onion flakes

¼ cup celery, chopped fine
2 tablespoons lemon juice
¼ teaspoon pepper
½ teaspoon salt or to taste
3 bay leaves

Combine all ingredients in Dutch oven. Simmer for 45 minutes. Water or additional tomato juice may be added if desired. Remove bay leaves before serving.

Celery and Potato Soup

4 cups celery, chopped
1 cup onion, chopped
½ cup Butter Buds Liquid
(see page 50)
1 clove garlic, minced
1¼ cups potatoes, peeled and
diced

¼ cup fresh parsley, chopped
4 cups chicken broth
½ teaspoon Beau Monde
seasoning
¼ teaspoon pepper

Sauté celery and onion in a non–stick Pam–sprayed skillet; add garlic, and sauté an additional minute. Stir in potatoes, Butter Buds Liquid, parsley and broth. Bring to a boil, cover, reduce heat and simmer 20 minutes. Pour half of soup mixture in electric blender and process until smooth; repeat. Stir in seasonings. Serve immediately.

Chicken Gumbo

3 cups onions, chopped
½ bunch green onions,
chopped
2 green peppers, chopped
1 rib celery, chopped
4 cups chicken broth
3 chicken bouillon cubes
2½ cups stewed tomatoes
1 teaspoon garlic
¼ cup fresh parsley, chopped
1 bay leaf

Salt and pepper to taste
3 tablespoons Fleischmann's
Fat Free Squeezable Spread
2½ pounds chicken breasts,
cooked and diced
1½ cups V–8 juice
1 (16–ounce) package frozen
cut okra
1 cup rice, cooked
1 tablespoon cornstarch
1 tablespoon water

Sauté onion, green onion, peppers and celery in a non–stick Pam–sprayed skillet. Transfer sautéed vegetables to a stock pot; add broth, bouillon, tomatoes, garlic, parsley, bay leaf, salt and pepper. Simmer for 45 minutes, covered. Add Fleischmann's, chicken and V–8 juice; simmer an additional 30 minutes. Add okra and rice; simmer 10 minutes. Make a paste using cornstarch and 1 tablespoon water. Add to soup mixture, stirring until slightly thickened.

Chicken & Rice Soup

8 cups chicken broth
1 carrot, diced small
1½ bay leaves
5 peppercorns
2 cups onions, diced
1 cup celery, diced

1 cup bell pepper, diced
1 teaspoon salt
¼ teaspoon pepper
½ cup Minute rice, uncooked
2 cups cooked chicken breast, chopped

Add first 9 ingredients. Simmer until carrots are tender. Add rice and chicken. Continue simmering for 1 hour.

Chicken Noodle Soup

6 cups water
6 chicken bouillon cubes
½ cup onions, diced
½ bay leaf
1 teaspoon salt
Pepper to taste
¾ teaspoon thyme

½ teaspoon parsley flakes
¼ cup celery, chopped
1¼ cups chicken breast, cooked and diced
3 cups yolkless egg noodles, cooked

Add all ingredients, omitting chicken and noodles. Bring slowly to a boil. Reduce heat; cover and simmer for 2 hours. Add cooked chicken and simmer an additional 30 to 45 minutes. Remove bay leaf before serving.

Corn Chowder

1 slice Oscar Mayer bacon
4 tablespoons onion, diced
1 quart skim milk
4 cups potatoes, peeled and diced

1 chicken bouillon cube
2½ cups cream style corn
1 tablespoon dried parsley
Salt and pepper to taste

In a Dutch oven add bacon, onion, milk, potatoes, bouillon cube, salt and pepper. Boil gently for 20 minutes or until potatoes are tender. Add corn and parsley. Bring to a gentle boil and cook an additional 10 minutes.

Chili con Carne

1 pound lean ground beef
2 cups onions, diced
½ teaspoon garlic powder
1 tablespoon chili powder
1½ cups water
3 teaspoons oregano
1 teaspoon paprika

2 pints tomatoes
2 cups kidney beans
¼ teaspoon cayenne pepper
½ tablespoon sugar
Salt to taste
Pepper to taste

Cook meat in a colander in the microwave; rinse. Combine all ingredients in a large saucepan. Heat to boiling; reduce heat to simmer, cooking for 2½ to 3 hours until consistency is to your desire.

Cream of Asparagus Soup

3 tablespoons Fleischmann's
Fat Free Squeezable Spread
1 tablespoon Ultra Promise
70% Less Fat
2 tablespoons flour
1 (14.5–ounce) can asparagus,
drained and liquid reserved

⅓ cup onion, finely chopped
and sautéed
4 chicken bouillon cubes
Water
Salt and pepper to taste

Mix Fleischmann's and Ultra Promise and flour until smooth. Add enough water to asparagus juice to make 4 cups; add bouillon and stir until dissolved. Gradually add bouillon mixture to flour and stir until smooth. Heat to boiling. Add sautéed onions and asparagus and simmer for 15 minutes. Cool slightly. Puree in small amounts in electric blender. Blend cream into soup. Add salt and pepper to taste. Heat to just boiling.

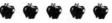

Cream of Broccoli Soup

1 cup water
1 (10–ounce) package frozen
  chopped broccoli
2 cups skim milk
2 cups fat–free Cheddar cheese,
  shredded
2 chicken bouillon cubes

½ cup flour
2 tablespoons Ultra Promise
  70% Less Fat
1 cup evaporated skimmed
  milk
Salt and pepper to taste

In a large saucepan, cook broccoli in 1 cup water. Do not drain. Place milk, cheese, bouillon, and flour into blender container. Cover and process at grind speed. Add evaporated milk, salt and pepper. Cook, stirring frequently, over medium heat until hot and mixture thickens.

Cream of Cucumber Soup

2 cups cucumbers, peeled and
  coarsely chopped
1 cup chicken broth
1 cup evaporated skimmed
  milk
¼ cup chives, chopped

¼ cup celery leaves, chopped
3 sprigs parsley
3 tablespoons Fleischmann's
  Fat Free Squeezable Spread
2 tablespoons flour
Salt to taste

Combine all ingredients in a blender; cover and blend until smooth. Serve hot or cold.

Cream of Red Pepper Soup

1 onion, finely chopped
2 cloves garlic, minced
4 red peppers, seeded and
  coarsely chopped
Juice and zest of 1 orange

6 cups vegetable stock
¼ cup sherry wine
Salt and pepper to taste
Chopped parsley

Sauté onion in a Pam–sprayed skillet; add garlic. Add peppers, orange juice and zest and cook over high heat until peppers are soft. Add stock; decrease heat and simmer for 15 to 20 minutes. Transfer soup to blender and puree. Return soup to pot and warm. Add sherry, salt and pepper. Ladle into soup bowls and garnish with chopped parsley.

Creamy Cauliflower Soup

2 (10–ounce) packages frozen
  cauliflower
½ cup onion, chopped
½ cup flour
2 cups water, divided
3 tablespoons Fleischmann's
  Fat Free Squeezable Spread
1½ tablespoons instant chicken
  bouillon

⅜ cup Kroger Lite Classics
  sharp Cheddar cheese
1½ cups fat–free Cheddar
  cheese, shredded
1 cup evaporated skimmed
  milk
1 cup skim milk

Cook cauliflower in 1 cup water until tender; drain, reserving liquid. Reserve 1 cup cauliflower and puree remaining cauliflower with reserved liquid. In a non–stick Pam–sprayed skillet, sauté onions. Make a paste of Fleischmann's and flour. Whisk 1 cup water with bouillon in flour paste. Heat bouillon mixture, stirring constantly until thickened. Stir in remaining ingredients. Cook until heated through.

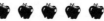

Crock Pot Stew

1 pound beef tenderloin, cut in
   1–inch cubes
¼ cup flour
½ teaspoon salt
½ teaspoon pepper
2½ cups beef broth
1 teaspoon Worcestershire
   sauce

1 clove garlic, minced
1 bay leaf
2 cups potatoes, peeled and
   diced
4 carrots, sliced
1 cup onion, diced
½ cup celery, sliced
2 teaspoons sugar

Place meat in crock pot. Mix flour, salt and pepper and pour over meat; stir to coat meat with flour. Add remaining ingredients and stir to mix well. Cover; cook on low 9 to 11 hours. (High 3 to 5 hours). Stir before serving.

Elegant French Onion Soup

5 cups yellow onions, thinly
   diced
1½ tablespoons Ultra Promise
   70% Less Fat
1½ tablespoons Fleischmann's
   Fat Free Squeezable Spread
1 teaspoon salt
1 teaspoon sugar

3 tablespoons flour
4 to 5 beef bouillon cubes
5¾ cups boiling water
½ cup dry white wine
⅛ teaspoon black pepper
Fat–free mozzarella cheese
1 cup croutons (see page 162)

Sauté onions in a Pam–sprayed Dutch oven. Adjust heat so that onions are thoroughly sautéed and have turned somewhat brown. (In order to achieve this, you may have to spray onions with Pam several times while cooking). Stir in salt and flour. In separate container mix bouillon with water. Add this immediately after stirring in flour. Add wine and pepper. Simmer partly covered for 30 minutes. Pour soup into individual bowls. Add cheese and croutons.

Field Pea Soup

1 cup onions, diced
3 cups fresh field peas (frozen may be used)
4 cups water
2 teaspoons basil
2 strips Oscar Mayer bacon
Salt and pepper to taste

Sauté onions in a Pam–sprayed non–stick skillet. Transfer to saucepan. Add peas, water, basil, salt, pepper and bacon. Simmer, covered, for 45 minutes to an hour. Remove bacon before serving.

Gazpacho

1 (32–ounce) can whole peeled tomatoes
1 tablespoon oregano
½ cup fresh bread crumbs
¼ cup red wine vinegar
1 cucumber, peeled and seeded
1 onion
1 clove garlic
1 green pepper, chopped

Place first 7 ingredients in blender until smooth. Garnish with green pepper. Serve chilled.

Hamburger and Lentil Soup

½ pound ground round
5¾ cups tomato juice
4 cups water
1 cup lentils
1 cup carrots, chopped
1 cup cabbage, chopped
1 cup celery, chopped
1 teaspoon salt
½ teaspoon pepper
½ green pepper, chopped
1 bay leaf
½ tablespoon parsley flakes

Cook ground round in colander in microwave, stirring occasionally, until done. In a Dutch oven, add all ingredients. Bring to a boil; reduce heat and simmer for 1½ hours. Remove bay leaf before serving.

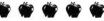

King Crab Stew

2½ cups fresh, canned or
   thawed frozen King
   crabmeat, in chunks,
   completely drained
2 tablespoons Ultra Promise
   70% Less Fat
3 tablespoons minced onion
1½ teaspoons salt

⅛ teaspoon pepper
¼ teaspoon dried rosemary
2½ cups skim milk
1 cup evaporated skimmed
   milk
2 tablespoons sherry
Dash Tabasco sauce
Chopped parsley

Remove cartilage from crabmeat, if canned. Melt Promise in top of a double boiler over direct heat. Add onion and cook until tender. Add crabmeat, salt, pepper and rosemary. Cook over low heat, stirring occasionally, for 8 minutes. Set double boiler top over boiling water; add milk and cook 15 minutes. Add evaporated skimmed milk. When hot, stir in sherry and Tabasco. Sprinkle with parsley and serve.

Lobster Bisque

2 cans Campbell's Healthy
   Request cream of mushroom
   soup
2 cans tomato soup, undiluted
⅔ cup dry sherry

1 cup evaporated skimmed
   milk
2½ cups skim milk
1 (5–ounce) can lobster meat
Salt and pepper to taste
Sliced green onion

Combine soups in a large saucepan; mix well. Stir in sherry, evaporated milk, and skim milk. Drain lobster; remove membrane. Add to soup mixture. Add salt and pepper. Bring just to boiling over medium heat, stirring occasionally. Ladle into soup cups. Garnish with green onion.

Manhattan Clam Chowder

1 pint clams
3 slices Oscar Mayer bacon,
  chopped
½ cup onion, chopped
½ cup green pepper, chopped
1 cup celery, chopped
1 cup clam liquor and water

1 cup potatoes, diced
¼ teaspoon thyme
½ teaspoon dried parsley
1 teaspoon salt
Dash cayenne pepper
2 cups tomato juice

Drain clams and save liquor; chop. Fry bacon until lightly brown; drain on paper towels. Sauté onions, peppers, and celery in a non–stick Pam–sprayed skillet. In a large pan, mix together onion mixture, clam liquor and water, potatoes, clam seasonings and clams. Cook for about 15 minutes or until potatoes are done. Add tomato juice; heat. Ladle into soup bowls and serve.

New England Clam Chowder

1 pint clams
3 slices Oscar Mayer bacon,
  chopped
¼ cup onion, chopped
1 cup clam liquor and water
1 cup potatoes, diced

½ teaspoon salt
Dash pepper
1 cup skim milk
1 cup evaporated skimmed
  milk
Green onions, chopped

Drain clams and save liquor; chop. Fry bacon until brown; drain on paper towels. Sauté onions in a non–stick Pam–sprayed skillet. In a large pan, combine onions, clam liquor, bacon, liquor and water, potatoes, seasoning and clams. Cook for about 15 minutes or until potatoes are done. Add milk; heat. Ladle into soup bowls and garnish with green onions.

Meatless Vegetable Soup

4 large carrots, sliced
2 medium potatoes, cubed
1 large onion, chopped
2½ cups celery, chopped
2 cups stewed tomatoes
1 small green pepper, chopped
1 teaspoon rosemary
1 teaspoon parsley flakes
1 bay leaf

½ teaspoon garlic powder
2 tablespoons Ultra Promise
   70% Less Fat
2 tablespoons Fleischmann's
   Fat Free Squeezable Spread
4 cups water
1 teaspoon sugar
Salt and pepper to taste

Combine all ingredients in Dutch oven. Simmer 2 to 3 hours. Add additional water or tomatoes to make desired consistency, if desired. Remove bay leaf before serving.

Ham & Cabbage Soup

4 cups chicken broth
1 cup Virginia ham, diced
   finely
3 onions, chopped
2 cups water
4 medium potatoes, peeled and
   cubed

1 small head cabbage,
   shredded
4 cups canned tomatoes
Salt and pepper to taste
Dash cayenne pepper

In a stock pot add broth, onions, water, potatoes, tomatoes and salt and pepper. Simmer slowly until vegetables are tender. Add ham, cabbage and cayenne pepper. Cook until cabbage is done.

Potato Soup

10 to 12 medium potatoes,
  peeled and diced
1 medium onion, chopped
1 teaspoon salt
6 cups water
4 chicken bouillon cubes

½ cup Ultra Promise Fat Free
1 (13–ounce) can evaporated
  skimmed milk
Pepper, to taste
Fat free Cheddar cheese,
  shredded

Combine potatoes, onion, salt and water in 4 quart saucepan. Bring to a boil; add bouillon cubes. Simmer until potatoes are tender. Add Promise and milk. Bring to a boil. Season with pepper and top with cheese.

Easy Corn Soup

1 can cream style corn
1½ cups evaporated skimmed
  milk
½ cup skim milk
3 chicken bouillon cubes
2 tablespoons Ultra Promise
  70% Less Fat

1 tablespoon Fleischmann's Fat
  Free Squeezable Spread
1 teaspoon fresh lemon juice
1 teaspoon marjoram
Salt and pepper to taste

Blend corn in blender. In a medium saucepan, combine all ingredients; bring to a boil, stirring constantly. Let simmer for 10 minutes. May be served hot or cold.

Lima Bean Soup

1 pound dried lima beans
3 quarts water
1 medium onion, finely
  chopped

1 stalk celery, finely chopped
4 tablespoons tomato paste
4 strips Oscar Mayer bacon
Salt and pepper to taste

Simmer beans and water in a large Dutch oven, until tender, about 1½ hours. Add onion, paste, celery, bacon, salt and pepper. Cook for another 45 minutes or until beans are well done. Stir frequently and add additional water if necessary. Remove bacon before serving.

Shrimp and Green Pepper Boil

2 cups chicken broth
4 cups canned diced tomatoes
  in juice
½ cup tomato puree
3 medium green peppers,
  chopped
1 onion, chopped
1 celery rib, chopped
½ pound frozen baby cooked
  shrimp

¼ cup rice, cooked
¼ cup cilantro, chopped
¼ cup green onions, chopped
Garlic to taste, chopped
Diced jalapeño pepper to taste
Salt to taste
Pinch of thyme
Pinch of saffron (optional)
1 bay leaf, crushed

Combine all ingredients in saucepan. Simmer until vegetables are tender. Serve hot.

Shrimp Chowder

2 slices Oscar Mayer bacon
½ cup onion, minced
1 (7–ounce) can shrimp
1 cup potatoes, chopped
1 can Campbell's Healthy
  Request cream of celery soup

1½ cups skim milk
1 (16–ounce) can cream style
  corn
Salt and pepper to taste

Cook bacon until crisp; drain, crumble and set aside. Sauté onions in a non–stick Pam–sprayed skillet. Drain shrimp, reserving liquid. Add shrimp liquid and potatoes to skillet. Cook, covered, over low heat for 15 minutes or until potatoes are tender. Add remaining ingredients; mix well. Heat to serving temperature; do not boil. Ladle into soup bowls.

Shrimp Gumbo

2 cups chicken bouillon
3 dozen medium–sized okra,
  sliced
1 cup onion
5 small tomatoes, peeled and
  coarsely chopped

2 tablespoons Ultra Promise
  70% Less Fat
Salt and pepper to taste
1 cup frozen salad shrimp,
  thawed
Rice, optional

Add bouillon, onion, tomatoes, Promise, salt and pepper; simmer 15 minutes. Add okra and shrimp. Cook until thick. May be served over rice.

Spinach and Garlic Soup

Garlic croutons (see page 161)
1 large bunch spinach, coarsely
  chopped
2 large carrots, grated
4 cups chicken bouillon
1 large onion, chopped
1 to 2 teaspoons garlic powder

1 tablespoons Butter Buds
  Powder
¼ cup flour
½ teaspoon salt
1 cup evaporated skimmed
  milk

Cook spinach and carrots in chicken broth until tender, about 10 minutes. Sauté onion in Pam–sprayed non–stick skillet. Add all ingredients, excluding the milk, in a blender. Process until smooth. Return to saucepan and add milk. Heat just to serving temperature. Serve with garlic croutons.

Split Pea Soup

1 box Reese green split peas
6 cups water
2 chicken bouillon cubes
1 onion, peeled and chopped
1 cup celery, chopped

1 cup evaporated skimmed
  milk
3 slices turkey ham ¼–inch
  thick, diced very small
Salt and pepper to taste

Combine peas, water, bouillon, onions, and celery in a Dutch oven. Bring almost to a boil. Reduce heat and gently simmer, covered, until done, about 2½ hours. Press through food mill. Return to Dutch oven; add milk, turkey ham, salt and pepper. Let simmer an additional 30 minutes.

Tomato Soup

2 cups onion, thinly sliced
1 teaspoon thyme
3 teaspoons basil
1 teaspoon garlic, or to taste
Salt and pepper to taste
½ cup Fleischmann's Fat Free
  Squeezable Spread

8 cups tomatoes, cored and
  diced
3 tablespoons tomato paste
¼ cup flour
4 cups chicken broth
1 teaspoon sugar
1 cup evaporated skimmed
  milk

Sauté onions in a Pam–sprayed non–stick 3 quart saucepan. Add thyme, basil, garlic, salt, pepper, Fleischmann's, tomatoes and tomato paste. Simmer for 15 minutes or until tomatoes are soft. Blend flour with 5 tablespoons broth in a small bowl. Stir into tomato mixture. Add remaining broth. Simmer for 30 minutes stirring frequently. Blend in a blender until smooth. Return to heat. Add sugar and evaporated milk. Heat to serving temperature.

Vegetable Beef Soup

½ pound lean Healthy Choice
  ground beef, cooked and
  drained
3 cups potatoes, diced
2 cups sliced carrots
1 medium onion, diced
1 package Lipton onion soup
1 (16–ounce) can pinto beans
1 (16–ounce) can stewed
  tomatoes
1 (5–ounce) frozen English
  peas
1 (10–ounce) box baby limas
1 (15–ounce) can whole kernel
  corn
1 tablespoon sugar
½ cup tomato sauce
Salt and pepper to taste

Cook potatoes, carrots, onion, and soup mix with just enough water that all is covered. Cook until tender. Then add baby limas and corn. Bring to a slow boil. Add remaining vegetables and cooked meat. Let simmer slowly for 2 to 3 hours.

Vegetarian Chili

1 envelope William's chili
  seasoning
1 (14½–ounce) can stewed
  tomatoes
1¼ cups water
Pinch of sugar
½ medium onion, chopped
1 (16–ounce) can black beans,
  drained and rinsed
1 (16–ounce) can dark red
  kidney beans, drained and
  rinsed
1 cup frozen whole kernel corn
2 zucchini, sliced

Combine first 5 ingredients in a Dutch oven. Simmer for 30 minutes. Add remaining ingredients and let simmer an additional 30 minutes.

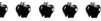

White Chili

½ pound ground turkey, cooked
½ cup onion, chopped
½ teaspoon garlic powder
3 cups water
2 (15–ounce) cans great Northern beans
1 (4–ounce) can green chili peppers
2 teaspoons chicken bouillon granules
1 teaspoon ground cumin
Salt to taste
¼ teaspoon white pepper
¼ cup water
2 tablespoons flour
1 cup fat–free mozzarella cheese, shredded

Cook turkey in colander in microwave. Sauté onions in Pam–sprayed skillet. Add onions and cooked turkey in saucepan along with the next 8 ingredients. Bring to a boil, reduce heat and simmer for 30 minutes. In a small bowl stir flour into ¼ cup water until there are no lumps. Add to chili. Cook and stir until thickened. Top servings with cheese.

White House Onion and Wine Soup

5 large onions
5 cups beef broth
½ cup celery leaves
1 large potato, peeled and sliced
2 tablespoons Ultra Promise 70% Less Fat
2 tablespoons Fleischmann's Fat Free Squeezable Spread
1 cup dry white wine
1 tablespoon vinegar
2 teaspoons sugar
1 cup evaporated skimmed milk
Salt and pepper to taste
Parmesan fat–free cheese

Sauté onions in a Pam–sprayed non–stick skillet until tender. Add beef broth, celery leaves and potato. Bring to a boil and cook 30 minutes, covered. Puree this mixture in blender. Return to saucepan. Add wine, vinegar and sugar. Bring to a boil. Simmer for 5 minutes. Stir in evaporated skimmed milk, Ultra Promise, Fleischmann's Fat Free Squeezable Spread, parsley, salt and pepper. Heat to serving temperature. Ladle into soup bowls and top with Parmesan cheese.

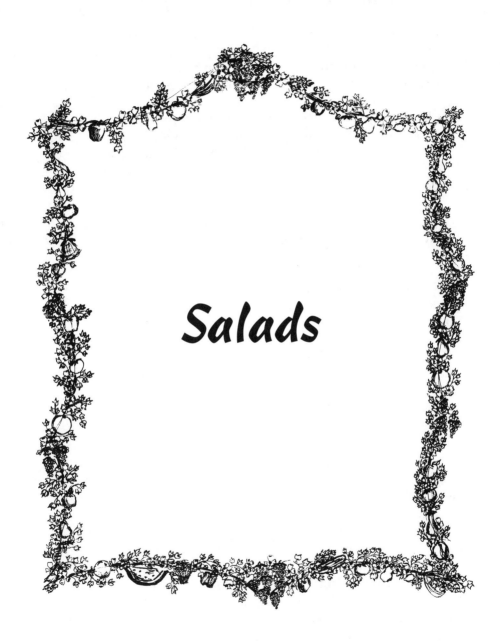

Salads

Aunt Jane's Summer Tomatoes

4 garden tomatoes, peeled and
  sliced
1 purple onion, peeled and
  thinly sliced

1 cup red wine vinegar
¾ cup water
⅛ cup sugar
1 tablespoon dried tarragon

Place layer of tomato slices alternately with layer of onion slices in
vegetable bowl. In separate bowl, combine vinegar, water and sugar;
stir until sugar is dissolved. Add tarragon and stir well. Pour over
slices and marinate in refrigerator at least 2 hours before serving,
basting at least every 30 minutes.

Beet Salad

1 can shoestring beets
1 (3–ounce) package lemon
  gelatin
¼ cup sugar

¼ cup vinegar
1 tablespoon prepared
  horseradish

Drain beets; reserve juice. Measure juice and add enough water to
make 1½ cups liquid. Bring to a boil; remove from heat. Add gelatin,
sugar, vinegar and horseradish. Stir until gelatin dissolves. Add
beets. Refrigerate until firm.

Black Bean Salad

1 can black beans, rinsed and
  drained
3 green onions, sliced
Zest of ½ lime, finely grated
½ tablespoon lime juice
1 teaspoon ground cumin
1 tablespoon frozen limeade
  concentrate, undiluted, or to
  taste

2 tablespoons green pepper,
  finely chopped
2 tablespoons red pepper,
  finely chopped
Fresh cilantro, chopped, to
  taste (optional)
Salt and pepper to taste

Combine all ingredients well. Refrigerate overnight to allow flavors
to blend.

Black-eyed Pea Salad

4 cups canned black-eyed peas,
   rinsed and drained
1 medium onion, finely
   chopped
2 ribs celery, finely chopped
1 small red pepper, finely
   chopped

1 garlic clove, crushed
¾ teaspoon dried basil
2 to 3 tablespoons cider vinegar
¼ teaspoon black pepper
1 teaspoon sugar
Salt to taste

In a medium bowl, combine peas, onion, celery and red pepper. In a separate bowl, combine garlic, basil, vinegar, pepper, sugar and salt; mix well. Pour vinegar mixture over pea mixture and toss gently. Refrigerate overnight.

Carrot-Apple Salad

2 cups carrots, shredded
1 cup apple, chopped
½ cup raisins

Weight Watcher's Fat Free
   Whipped Dressing

Mix first 3 ingredients. Add enough whipped dressing to light coat the ingredients. Refrigerate.

Chilled Tomato Mold

1 can Campbell's tomato soup
2 envelopes unflavored gelatin
1 cup fat-free cottage cheese,
   drained

½ cup celery, finely chopped
½ cup cucumbers, finely
   chopped
½ tablespoon parsley flakes

Sprinkle gelatin over soup and let stand 5 minutes. Add other ingredients and pour into mold. Chill until set.

Chinese Pea Pod Salad

2 (10–ounce) boxes frozen
   Chinese pea pods, thawed
8 ounces fresh mushrooms,
   sliced
2 pints cherry tomatoes, halved

1 red onion, sliced
½ yellow pepper, sliced
Italian fat–free dressing
Fat–free Parmesan cheese

Mix first 5 ingredients in salad bowl. Add enough Italian dressing to lightly coat vegetables. Sprinkle with Parmesan cheese. Toss gently. Serve immediately.

Cissy's Freezer Slaw

1 medium head cabbage,
   shredded
1 teaspoon salt
1 carrot, grated
1 green pepper, chopped

1 cup white vinegar
¼ cup water
2 cups sugar
1 teaspoon whole mustard seed
1 teaspoon celery seed

Mix cabbage and salt in bowl and let stand 1 hour. Add carrot and green pepper. Combine next 5 ingredients in a saucepan. Boil for 1 minute. Cool to lukewarm. Pour over slaw. Spoon into freezer containers. Store in freezer.

Cole Slaw

3 cups shredded cabbage
1 cup shredded carrots

½ cup + 2 tablespoons Weight
   Watcher's Fat Free Whipped
   Dressing
½ tablespoon vinegar

Mix all ingredients; chill before serving.

Congealed Asparagus

1½ cups cold water, divided
½ cup white vinegar
¾ cup sugar
½ teaspoon salt
2½ envelopes unflavored
gelatin
1 tablespoon lemon juice

1 (10½–ounce) can asparagus
spears, drained
1 (2–ounce) jar pimentos,
drained
¾ cup celery, finely chopped
1 teaspoon grated onion
3 egg whites, boiled and diced

Heat 1 cup water and vinegar to boiling. Add sugar and salt, stirring until dissolved. Mix gelatin in ½ cup water. Add to hot mixture and stir until gelatin mixture completely dissolves. Chill until gelatin mixture is slightly thickened. Add remaining ingredients. Pour into Pam–sprayed mold. Chill until firm.

Congealed Spinach Salad

1 (3–ounce) package lime
gelatin
1 cup boiling water
1 (10–ounce) package frozen
chopped spinach, thawed and
squeezed dry
1 cup Weight Watcher's Fat
Free Whipped Dressing

1 cup fat–free cottage cheese,
drained
¼ teaspoon wine vinegar
½ cup fresh parsley, chopped
1 teaspoon onion, grated
1 teaspoon fresh lemon juice

Dissolve gelatin in boiling water. Stir in remaining ingredients in order listed. Pour into a Pam–sprayed 9 x 9–inch pan. Chill until firm.

Creamy Carrot Salad

1 (3–ounce) package orange
  gelatin
1 cup boiling water
⅜ cup fat–free sour cream
⅛ cup Weight Watcher's Fat
  Free Whipped Dressing

1 (8½–ounce) can crushed
  pineapple, undrained
¼ cup golden raisins
1 cup carrots, finely shredded

Pour boiling water over gelatin, stirring until dissolved. Spoon whipped dressing into a bowl with sour cream. Gradually add gelatin mixture, stirring until blended. Chill until mixture begins to thicken. Stir in remaining ingredients. Turn into a Pam–sprayed mold. Refrigerate until set.

Creamy Cucumber and Tomatoes

2 medium cucumbers
2 green onions, chopped
1 teaspoon salt
1½ cups tomatoes, chopped
2 teaspoons dried cilantro

½ teaspoon ground cumin
⅛ teaspoon black pepper
½ clove garlic, finely chopped
1 cup fat–free sour cream

Cut cucumbers in half lengthwise and scoop out seeds; chop. Mix cucumbers, onions and salt in large bowl; let stand 10 minutes. Stir in tomatoes and seasonings. Cover and refrigerate for 1 hour or until chilled. Drain thoroughly. Just before serving, fold in sour cream.

Crunchy Citrus Broccoli

4 cups broccoli flowerets
1 small purple onion, chopped
½ cup raisins
1 (11–ounce) can mandarin
  oranges, drained

1 cup Weight Watcher's Fat
  Free Whipped Dressing
¼ cup sugar

Mix together whipped dressing and sugar. Mix remaining ingredients. Gently toss with dressing. Marinate overnight. Serve cold.

Curried Potato Salad

4 medium potatoes, diced
½ cup fat–free French dressing
1 teaspoon salt
Pepper to taste
¾ cup celery, finely chopped
¼ cup onion, chopped
3 egg whites, hard–boiled and
  diced

¼ cup sweet pickle relish
½ cup Weight Watcher's Fat
  Free Whipped Dressing
½ teaspoon curry
2 teaspoons parsley flakes
Paprika

Cook potatoes in salted water until done; drain well. While still warm toss with French dressing, salt and pepper. Let stand for about 2 hours. Add celery, onion, eggs, relish, curry and parsley. Add whipped dressing and toss gently. Sprinkle top with paprika.

Debbie's Stuffed Garden Tomatoes

Garden tomatoes
Fat–free cottage cheese
Cucumbers, peeled and diced
Green onions, sliced
Weight Watcher's Fat Free
  Whipped Dressing

Black pepper
Lawry's seasoned salt
Paprika
Parsley

Wash tomatoes. Hollow tomatoes with a spoon. Pepper and season salt inside of tomatoes. Combine cottage cheese, cucumbers, and onions. Use just enough whipped dressing to taste. Fill tomato cavity with cottage cheese mixture; chill. Before serving, sprinkle tops with paprika and a sprig of parsley.

Dee Dee's Broccoli Salad

1 head of broccoli, cut up
White raisins
Green onions, chopped
½ cup fat–free Cheddar cheese,
  shredded

Jennie–O turkey bacon, cooked
  and crumbled
1 cup Weight Watcher's Fat
  Free Whipped Dressing
2 tablespoons vinegar
½ cup sugar

Cook turkey bacon in microwave, crumble and set aside. Mix together whipped dressing, vinegar and sugar; set aside. Combine broccoli, raisins, onions and cheese. Toss with dressing mixture. Refrigerate overnight. Just before serving, stir in bacon.

Deviled Eggs

12 hard–boiled eggs, halved,
  and yolks discarded
1 cup Egg Beaters
½ cup Weight Watcher's Fat
  Free Whipped Dressing

⅓ cup sweet pickle relish
2 teaspoons prepared mustard
Salt and pepper to taste
Paprika for garnish

Cook Egg Beaters according to microwave directions for scrambled eggs. Mash until the consistency of cooked, mashed egg yolks. Add remaining ingredients. Spoon Egg Beater mixture into egg whites. Sprinkle with paprika.

English Pea Salad

1 (#2) can English peas, drained
4 tablespoons Weight
  Watcher's Fat Free Whipped
  Dressing

2 egg whites, boiled and diced
¼ cup fat–free Cheddar cheese
1 tablespoon pimento
Salt and pepper to taste

Mix all ingredients. Refrigerate overnight to allow flavors to blend.

Fresh Broccoli & Cauliflower Salad

DRESSING:

1 cup Weight Watcher's Fat
   Free Whipped Dressing

2 tablespoons sugar
2 tablespoons vinegar

Mix the above ingredients well.

SALAD:

1 bunch broccoli, chopped
1 small head cauliflower,
   chopped
½ cup purple onion, chopped

1 cup white raisins
3 slices Oscar Mayer bacon,
   cooked crisp and crumbled

Mix all ingredients. Add dressing and refrigerate overnight.

Fancy Macaroni Salad

8 ounces macaroni
1 cup celery, diced
½ cup green onions, sliced
¼ cup radishes, thinly sliced
2 teaspoons parsley flakes
½ cup Weight Watcher's Fat
   Free Whipped Dressing

½ cup fat–free sour cream
2 tablespoons white vinegar
1 teaspoon lemon juice
2 teaspoons prepared mustard
2 teaspoons salt
⅛ teaspoon pepper

Cook macaroni according to directions; drain well. Rinse in cold water; drain again. Add celery, onions and radishes. Sprinkle with parsley. In a separate bowl, combine remaining ingredients. Pour this over macaroni mixture and toss well. Refrigerate several hours before serving.

Garden Couscous

2 cups tomatoes, chopped
½ cup red pepper, finely
  chopped
8 green onions, chopped
1 (15–ounce) can garbanzo
  beans, rinsed and drained

1 teaspoon dried oregano
1 teaspoon paprika
1 clove garlic, finely chopped
5 cups couscous, cooked and
  hot
¼ cup fat–free Parmesan cheese

Combine first 7 ingredients in a 2–quart saucepan. Heat to boiling, stirring frequently. Serve over hot couscous and top with cheese.

Garden Fresh Vegetable Toss

3 fresh tomatoes, sliced
1 Bermuda onion, sliced
1 cucumber, peeled and sliced
1 green pepper, sliced
1 yellow pepper, sliced
½ cup vinegar

2 tablespoons red wine
2 tablespoons sugar
¼ teaspoon salt
¼ teaspoon basil
¼ teaspoon parsley flakes
Pepper to taste

Slice vegetables and put in a bowl. In separate bowl combine remaining ingredients. Pour over vegetables. Cover and let marinate overnight. Refrigerate.

Kidney Bean Toss

1 (16–ounce) can kidney beans,
  rinsed and drained
1 onion, chopped
2 tablespoons pickle relish
1 tablespoon pimento
½ teaspoon mustard

½ teaspoon salt
Pepper to taste
2 egg whites, boiled and diced
Weight Watcher's Fat Free
  Whipped Dressing

Combine all ingredients with enough whipped dressing to hold together. Refrigerate for several hours allowing flavors to blend.

Kraut Salad

1 quart sauerkraut
½ cup celery, chopped
½ cup green onions, bottoms
   only, sliced

1½ cups sugar
½ cup vinegar

Bring sugar and vinegar to a boil; let cool. Mix together sauerkraut, celery and onions. Pour vinegar mixture over vegetables.

Lettuce Slaw

1 head lettuce
½ cup cider vinegar
2 tablespoons sugar
1 tablespoon flour
½ teaspoon dry mustard

¼ teaspoon salt
⅛ teaspoon pepper
2 Egg Beaters
2 tablespoons evaporated
   skimmed milk

Core, rinse and drain lettuce. Tear into small pieces; set aside and refrigerate. Heat vinegar to boiling. In separate bowl, combine sugar, flour, mustard, salt and pepper. Add Egg Beaters and beat just until blended. Stir in a little of the hot vinegar, then add mixture to remaining vinegar. Cook over low heat, stirring constantly until thickened, about 5 minutes. Stir in milk; chill. Toss dressing and lettuce well just before serving.

Mayonnaise Potato Salad

4 cups potatoes, peeled, diced,
   cooked and drained
¼ cup sweet pickle relish
¼ onion, diced

4 eggs, boiled, diced and yolks
   discarded
4 heaping tablespoons Weight
   Watcher's Fat Free Whipped
   Dressing

In a medium bowl, mix together all ingredients. Keep chilled.

Macaroni Salad I

1 (8–ounce) package elbow
    macaroni
1 cup celery, chopped
⅛ cup fresh parsley, chopped
⅓ cup green pepper, chopped
6 green onions, sliced
2 egg whites, boiled and
    chopped
1 (2–ounce) jar pimento,
    drained

½ cup Weight Watcher's Fat
    Free Whipped Dressing
½ cup fat–free sour cream
1 tablespoon red wine vinegar
¼ teaspoon seasoned salt
¼ teaspoon pepper
⅔ cup fat–free Cheddar cheese,
    shredded

Cook macaroni according to package directions; drain and cool by running cold water over macaroni; drain well. Add next 6 ingredients and stir gently. In a separate bowl, mix together next 5 ingredients; mix well.

Pour dressing over macaroni mixture and gently toss. Cover and chill at least 2 hours. Before serving, toss with shredded cheese.

Macaroni Salad II

1 package tiny salad macaroni
    rings
4 egg whites, hard boiled and
    diced
1 (13–ounce) can tuna
1 cup celery, finely chopped
¼ cup onion, finely chopped

1 (17–ounce) can LeSeur
    English peas, drained
4 ounces fat–free Cheddar
    cheese, shredded
1 (2–ounce) jar pimentos
Salt and pepper to taste

Cook macaroni. Chill under cold running water and drain. Mix all ingredients together, tossing well.

DRESSING:
¼ cup Weight Watcher's Fat
    Free Whipped Dressing

1 tablespoon mustard

Mix well and toss with macaroni mixture.

Mixed Vegetable Salad

1 (10–ounce) package frozen
  English peas, thawed
1 cup celery, finely chopped
1 small cauliflower, wash and
  separate flowerets

1 small package radishes, diced
1 bunch green onions, sliced
1 (2–ounce) jar pimentos
¾ cup Weight Watcher's Fat
  Free Whipped Dressing

Mix all ingredients together thoroughly. Refrigerate for several hours allowing flavors to blend.

Overnight Pasta Salad

1 cup seashell pasta
2 cups lettuce, shredded
3 hard boiled eggs, yellows
  discarded, chopped
1 cup turkey ham, ½–inch
  cubed

1 (10–ounce) package tiny
  frozen peas, thawed
1 cup fat–free mozzarella
  cheese, shredded

DRESSING:
½ cup Weight Watcher's Fat
  Free Whipped Dressing
¼ cup fat–free sour cream
1 tablespoon cider vinegar

¼ cup green onions, thinly
  diced
1 teaspoon Dijon mustard
Dash Tabasco

Cook seashells according to package directions. Place lettuce in the bottom of glass salad bowl. Top with seashells, eggs, turkey ham, peas and cheese, in that order. In a small mixing bowl, combine remaining ingredients. Spread over top of salad, sealing to edge of bowl. Cover and refrigerate overnight. Toss before serving.

Pea Salad

2 (10–ounce) packages green
  peas, thawed
1½ cups fat–free sour cream
1 teaspoon soy sauce
Dash garlic salt

Dash onion salt
Dash pepper
2 teaspoons Worcestershire
  sauce
Purple onion, chopped, to taste

Steam thawed peas for 1 minute and then cool. Add remaining
ingredients. Refrigerate overnight to allow flavors to blend.

Springtime Salad

1 head lettuce, broken into
  bite–sized pieces
1 head cauliflower, cut into
  flowerets
1 large purple onion, sliced
8 slices Jennie–O turkey bacon,
  cooked and crumbled

3 tablespoons sugar
4 tablespoons fat–free
  Parmesan cheese
1 cup Weight Watcher's Fat
  Free Whipped Dressing
Salt and pepper to taste

Layer vegetables in glass salad bowl. In separate bowl mix together
sugar, whipped dressing, salt and pepper. Top vegetables with
dressing mixture. Sprinkle top with Parmesan cheese. Refrigerate
overnight. Sprinkle top with bacon before serving.

Summer Corn Salad

1 (#2) can shoepeg white corn,
  drained
3 green onions, sliced
1 small green pepper, chopped
1 cup celery, finely chopped
½ cup Weight Watcher's Fat
  Free Whipped Dressing

1 tablespoon prepared
  horseradish mustard
1 tablespoon lemon juice
Salt to taste
White pepper to taste
1 tablespoon pimento

Combine whipped dressing, mustard and lemon juice. In separate
bowl, combine remaining ingredients. Toss with whipped dressing
mixture. Refrigerate overnight.

Summer Potato Salad

4 cups potatoes, peeled, diced,
   cooked and drained
¼ cup sweet pickle relish
¼ cup onion, finely diced

4 eggs, boiled, diced and yolks
   discarded
¼ cup mustard
¼ cup Weight Watcher's Fat
   Free Whipped Dressing

In a medium bowl, mix all ingredients together. Keep chilled.

Tarragon Potato Salad

4 cups potatoes, peeled, diced,
   cooked and drained
¼ cup celery, finely chopped
⅛ cup green pepper, finely
   chopped
⅛ cup purple onion, finely
   chopped

½ cup fat free sour cream
½ cup Weight Watcher's Fat
   Free Whipped Dressing
1 teaspoon dried tarragon
1 tablespoon tarragon vinegar
Salt and pepper to taste

Mix together first 4 ingredients. In a separate bowl, mix sour cream, whipped dressing, tarragon and vinegar. Fold this into potato mixture. Refrigerate several hours so that flavors can blend. Keep refrigerated.

Tossed Corn Salad

2 (12–ounce) cans white whole
   kernel corn
1 medium cucumber, diced
1 medium onion, diced
1 large tomato, diced
½ cup fat–free sour cream

¼ cup Weight Watcher's Fat
   Free Whipped Dressing
2 tablespoons white vinegar
1 teaspoon salt
½ teaspoon dry mustard
½ teaspoon celery salt
½ teaspoon white pepper

Drain corn. Mix together all ingredients. Refrigerate overnight allowing flavors to blend.

Tomato Aspic Ring

1¼ cups tomato juice	3 tablespoons vinegar
1 cup water	1 tablespoon prepared
2 (3–ounce) packages lemon	horseradish
gelatin	1 teaspoon onion salt
1 cup fat–free sour cream	1 teaspoon sugar
1 cup Weight Watcher's Fat	4 drops Tabasco
Free Whipped Dressing	

Heat tomato juice almost to boiling. Pour over gelatin and stir until gelatin dissolves completely. Cool until syrupy but not set. Add remaining ingredients and beat until smooth. Pour into 5–cup ring mold rinsed with cold water. Cover and chill until firm. Unmold on a bed of lettuce.

Vegetable Pasta Toss

8 ounces corkscrew shaped	1 (10–ounce) package frozen
pasta	mixed vegetables
1 cup fat–free Italian dressing	1 teaspoon basil
¼ teaspoon green pepper	3 tablespoons green onions
	1 cup cherry tomatoes, halved

Cook pasta according to package directions. Place hot pasta in bowl and toss with salad dressing and pepper. Add frozen mixed vegetables and toss again. Add green onions. Just before serving add cherry tomato halves. Serve chilled.

Apple–Date Delight

8 apples	1 teaspoon cinnamon
1 cup chopped dates	½ teaspoon nutmeg
½ cup brown sugar, packed	Dash of salt

Core apples and slice. Add remaining ingredients. Pour into a Pam–sprayed casserole dish; cover. Bake at 350° for 40 minutes then uncover. Bake an additional 15 to 20 minutes.

Apricot Salad

1 (3–ounce) box orange gelatin
1 (3–ounce) box lemon gelatin
2 cups boiling water
½ teaspoon salt
1 teaspoon vinegar

2 tablespoons Weight
Watcher's Fat Free Whipped
Dressing
1 cup fat–free sour cream
1 small can crushed pineapple
1 small can apricots, chopped

Pour boiling water over gelatin; stir to dissolve. Let cool. Add remaining ingredients. Refrigerate until firm.

Apricot–Orange Mold

2 (16–ounce) cans apricot
halves
2 (3–ounce) packages orange
gelatin
2 tablespoons lemon juice

1 (6–ounce) can frozen orange
juice concentrate
1 cup lemon–lime carbonated
beverage, chilled
1 tablespoon orange rind,
grated

Drain apricots, reserving 1½ cups syrup. Puree apricots. Heat reserved syrup to boiling. Dissolve gelatin in syrup. Add puree, orange juice concentrate, lemon juice and orange rind. Stir until juice is dissolved. Slowly pour beverage down side of pan and mix gently. Pour into ring mold and chill. To serve, slice and top with Lemon Dressing.

LEMON DRESSING:
1 Egg Beater
½ cup sugar
2 tablespoons lemon juice
1 tablespoon lemon peel

1½ cups Dream Whip, prepared
(see page 329), or Cool Whip
Free

Mix first 4 ingredients and cook on medium heat until thick, about 5 minutes. Cool mixture and fold in Dream Whip or Cool Whip.

Bing Cherry Salad

1 (3–ounce) package red cherry
   gelatin
1 cup juice from cherries and
   pineapple
¼ cup Bing cherries, drained

¼ cup crushed pineapple,
   drained
4 ounces fat–free cream cheese
1 small coke
1 cup miniature marshmallows

Heat fruit juices and stir in gelatin. Chill until begins to thicken. Mix in cream cheese. Fold in fruit and coke until completely mixed. Chill until firm.

Blackberry Salad

1 (#2) can crushed pineapple,
   drained
1 (6–ounce) package blackberry
   jello
1 (#2) can blackberries, drained
2 cups hot water

1 ounce fat–free cream cheese
1½ cups fat–free sour cream
½ cup sugar
1 teaspoon vanilla
1 teaspoon lemon juice

Dissolve jello in water; add pineapple and blackberries. Refrigerate overnight. Next day combine remaining ingredients, blending thoroughly. Place on top of jello mixture. Keep refrigerated.

Blueberry Salad

2 cups boiling water
1 (3–ounce) package grape
   gelatin
½ cup pineapple, diced

1½ cups blueberry pie filling
1½ cups fat–free sour cream
½ cup sugar

Dissolve gelatin in boiling water. Add sugar. Let cool. Add sour cream; mix well. Add pineapple and pie filling. Cover and refrigerate until set.

Blueberry Salad with Topping

2 (3–ounce) boxes blackberry
    gelatin
2 cups boiling water
1 (15–ounce) can blueberries
1 (8–ounce) can crushed
    pineapple

1 (8–ounce) package fat–free
    cream cheese
1 cup fat–free sour cream
½ cup sugar
½ teaspoon vanilla extract

Drain fruit and reserve 1 cup total. Dissolve gelatin in boiling water. Add reserved fruit juice. Allow to cool. Add drained fruit. Pour into a 2–quart dish. Cover and refrigerate until firm. Combine cream cheese, sour cream, sugar and extract. Top salad with cream cheese mixture.

Camille's Lime Jello

1 (3–ounce) package lime
    gelatin
1¼ cups hot water
1 cup pineapple, drained

2 tablespoons horseradish
½ cup Weight Watcher's Fat
    Free Whipped Dressing
1 cup fat–free cottage cheese

Dissolve gelatin in hot water. Let partially set. Stir in remaining ingredients. Chill until firm.

Cherry Salad

1 (6–ounce) package raspberry
    gelatin
2 cups boiling water

2 (#2) cans dark red sweet
    pitted cherries
2 tablespoons reduced fat
    peanut butter

Dissolve gelatin in the boiling water. Add peanut butter and mix well. Add cherries and juice. Pour into serving dish; cover and chill.

Candied Apple Salad

1 cup water
¼ cup cinnamon candies
1 (3–ounce) package lemon
  gelatin
1 (#2) can applesauce

1 (8–ounce) package fat–free
  cream cheese
½ cup Weight Watcher's Fat
  Free Whipped Dressing
1 tablespoon confectioners
  sugar

Combine water and candies in saucepan; heat to boiling. Simmer, stirring occasionally, until candies are melted. Add gelatin; stir until dissolved. Add applesauce; mix well. Pour half of mixture into pan; chill until firm. Beat cream cheese, whipped dressing and sugar. Spread evenly over congealed mixture. Pour remaining gelatin mixture over cream cheese mixture. Chill until firm.

Chilled Minted Fruit

½ cup sugar
¾ cup water
2 tablespoons fresh lime juice
1 teaspoon fresh mint, chopped
Dash of salt

5 cups fresh cantaloupe, sliced
  or diced
4 cups fresh peaches, sliced or
  diced
2 cups fresh blueberries
1 cup fresh grapes

Combine first 5 ingredients in a small saucepan. Bring to a boil for 2 minutes. Cover; steep for 10 minutes. Strain syrup over prepared fruit. Cover; chill for at least 2 hours before serving.

Crunchy Salad

1 (3–ounce) package peach
  gelatin
1 cup boiling water

1 cup applesauce
½ cup carrots, finely grated
¼ cup celery, finely chopped

Dissolve gelatin in water. Add remaining ingredients. Chill until firm.

Congealed Blueberry Salad

1 (16–ounce) can blueberries, drained, with juice reserved
1 (8½–ounce) can crushed pineapple, drained, with juice reserved
1 (3–ounce) package black cherry gelatin

1 (3–ounce) package raspberry gelatin
2 cups boiling water
1 (8–ounce) package fat–free cream cheese
½ cup sugar
1 cup fat–free sour cream
½ teaspoon vanilla extract

Dissolve gelatins in boiling water. Add 1 cup pineapple and blueberry juice combined to gelatin. Stir in drained fruit. Pour into 9 x 13–inch dish to congeal. Mix together remaining ingredients and top congealed salad. Refrigerate.

Congealed Banana Salad

1 (6–ounce) package lemon gelatin
1½ cups boiling water
1½ cups miniature marshmallows
1 (#2) can crushed pineapple
3 bananas, sliced
½ cup sugar
1½ tablespoons flour

1 Egg Beater
1 teaspoon lemon peel, freshly grated
1 package Dream Whip, prepared (see page 329), or Cool Whip Free
2 cups fat–free Cheddar cheese, shredded

Dissolve gelatin in water. Add marshmallows. Drain pineapple and reserve liquid. Stir pineapple and bananas in gelatin. Refrigerate until firm. Cook pineapple juice, sugar, flour, Egg Beater and peel until thick. Cool. Fold in Dream Whip or Cool Whip. Spoon over gelatin mixture. Top with cheese before serving.

Cranberry Salad I

2 (3–ounce) packages
  strawberry gelatin
2½ cups boiling water
2 cups cranberries, raw

1 large seedless orange
2 large apples, cored
½ cup crushed pineapple

Dissolve gelatin in the boiling water. Grate cranberries, orange and apples. Add to gelatin mixture. Add sugar and pineapple. Stir well. Chill until firm.

Cranberry Salad II

2 (3–ounce) packages raspberry
  gelatin
2 cups boiling water
1 cup port wine
1 (#2) can crushed pineapple,
  undrained
1 (#2) can whole cranberry
  sauce

½ cup white grapes, halved
1 cup celery, finely chopped
1 (8–ounce) package fat–free
  cream cheese
⅓ cup Weight Watcher's Fat
  Free Whipped Dressing

Dissolve gelatin in the boiling water; cool slightly. Add wine; chill until partially congealed. Stir in next four ingredients. Cover; chill until firm. In a separate bowl, blend together cream cheese and whipped dressing. Spread cream cheese mixture on top. Chill and serve.

Creamy Cherry Salad

1 (#2) can cherry pie filling
1 can fat–free Eagle Brand milk
1 (9–ounce) can crushed
  pineapple, drained
1 (8–ounce) carton fat–free sour
  cream

4 cups Dream Whip, prepared
  (see page 329), or Cool Whip
  Free
1 tablespoon lemon juice

Mix together first 4 ingredients. Fold in Dream Whip or Cool Whip and lemon juice. Refrigerate until set.

Creamy Cranberry Salad

6 ounces fat–free cream cheese
2 tablespoons Weight Watcher's Fat Free Whipped Dressing
2 tablespoons sugar
1 (#2) can whole cranberry sauce
1 (9–ounce) can crushed pineapple, drained
1 cup Dream Whip, prepared (see page 329), or Cool Whip Free

Beat cream cheese; add dressing and sugar. Add pineapple then cranberry sauce, mixing thoroughly. Fold in Dream Whip or Cool Whip. Freeze. To serve, let stand for 10 minutes. Slice and serve on lettuce leaves.

Crunchy Fruit Salad

1 cup apple, chopped
1 (8–ounce) can pineapple chunks, drained
¼ cup celery, finely chopped
½ cup raisins
1 cup bananas, sliced
⅓ cup Weight Watcher's Fat Free Whipped Dressing
1 tablespoon fresh lemon juice

Chop apple and toss with lemon juice. Add remaining ingredients omitting banana. Chill for at least 1 hour. Add banana just before serving.

Frosty Grape Salad

6 ounces fat–free cream cheese
2 tablespoons Weight Watcher's Fat Free Whipped Dressing
1 (#2) can crushed pineapple, reserving 2 tablespoons juice
24 marshmallows, cut up
1 cup Dream Whip, prepared (see page 329), or Cool Whip Free
2 cups seedless grapes, chopped

Combine cream cheese and whipped dressing; beat until smooth. Beat in pineapple juice. Add marshmallows and pineapple. Fold in Dream Whip or Cool Whip and grapes. Pour into a 1 quart container; cover and freeze.

Frozen Cranberry Salad

1 (16–ounce) can cranberry
  sauce
3 tablespoons lemon juice
1 cup Dream Whip, prepared
  (see page 329), or Cool Whip
  Free

¼ cup Weight Watcher's Fat
  Free Whipped Dressing
⅛ cup confectioners sugar

Crush cranberry sauce with a fork. Add lemon juice. Pour into an aluminum foil muffin tin. Combine remaining ingredients; spread over cranberry mixture. Freeze.

Frozen Creamy Fruit Salad

¾ cup sugar
⅛ teaspoon salt
2 tablespoons lemon juice
1 pint fat–free sour cream

2 large bananas, mashed
¼ cup cherries, chopped
1 (9–ounce) can crushed
  pineapple, drained

Mix sour cream, lemon juice, sugar and salt. Add remaining ingredients and stir until evenly blended. Pour into aluminum foil tins which have been placed in muffin tins. Place in freezer for at least 4 hours.

Frozen Fruit Salad I

1 (8–ounce) package fat–free
  cream cheese
1 banana, mashed
½ cup frozen, sweetened
  strawberries, thawed
½ cup pineapple, crushed,
  drained

¼ cup sugar
2 cups Dream Whip, prepared
  (see page 329), or Cool Whip
  Free
2 drops red food coloring

Soften cream cheese and add next 4 ingredients, mixing well after each addition. Add food coloring. Fold Dream Whip or Cool Whip into cream cheese mixture. Pour into aluminum foil baking cups. Freeze. Serve with dollop of Dream Whip or Cool Whip Free or fat–free sour cream.

Frozen Fruit Salad II

1 (8–ounce) package fat–free
   cream cheese
½ cup Weight Watcher's Fat
   Free Whipped Dressing
1 (#2) can fruit cocktail
1 (6–ounce) jar cherries, halved
1 cup small marshmallows

1 (11–ounce) can mandarin
   oranges
½ teaspoon allspice
1 cup Dream Whip, prepared
   (see page 329), or Cool Whip
   Free

Soften cream cheese and blend with whipped dressing. Drain all fruit. Add allspice, marshmallows and fruit, mixing well. Fold Dream Whip or Cool Whip Free into mixture. Pour into freezable container and freeze.

Frozen Salad

25 large marshmallows,
   quartered
1 (#2) can crushed pineapple,
   drained, juice reserved
1 (10–ounce) jar maraschino
   cherries, halved, juice reserved

1 (8–ounce) package fat–free
   cream cheese
1 cup Dream Whip, prepared
   (see page 329), or Cool Whip
   Free

Combine quartered marshmallows, pineapple and drained cherries into a bowl. Let stand at room temperature for 2 hours. Mix cherry juice and cream cheese until thoroughly blended. Drain juice from pineapple mixture and add to cream cheese mixture until blended. Add pineapple mixture, mixing well. Fold in Dream Whip or Cool Whip Free. Pour into freezable container; cover and freeze.

Frozen Strawberry Salad

1 (3–ounce) package strawberry
   gelatin

1¼ cups hot water
1 pint vanilla fat–free ice cream
1 cup strawberries, diced small

Dissolve gelatin in hot water. Spoon in ice cream and stir until melted. Place in refrigerator for 20 minutes or until slightly thickened. Fold in strawberries. Freeze for 1 hour before serving.

Fruit Delight

1 (#2) can sliced peaches, cut
   into bite sizes
1 (#2) can fruit cocktail
1 (#2) can pineapple chunks
5 bananas, sliced

1 (6–ounce) jar maraschino
   cherries, drained and halved
1 (3.4–ounce) package lemon
   instant pudding
1 (3.4–ounce) package vanilla
   instant pudding

Mix undrained peaches, fruit cocktail, and pineapple chunks with drained cherries in a large mixing bowl. Add dry pudding mixes and stir. Chill thoroughly. Just before serving, add sliced bananas and toss.

Fruit Mold Salad

1 (3–ounce) package orange–
   pineapple gelatin
1 tablespoon sugar
1 cup boiling water
¾ cup cold water
1 cup Dream Whip, prepared
   (see page 329), or Cool Whip
   Free

¾ cup mandarin orange
   sections
1¼ cups seeded red grapes,
   halved
1 banana, sliced

Dissolve gelatin and sugar in boiling water. Add cold water. Chill until slightly thickened. Fold in Dream Whip or Cool Whip Free, then remaining ingredients. Pour into large mold. Chill until firm.

Fruit Salad Surprise

16 large marshmallows
1 (20–ounce) can pineapple
   tidbits, drained, reserving 2
   tablespoons juice

1 (8–ounce) package fat–free
   cream cheese, room
   temperature
1 (20–ounce) can fruit cocktail,
   drained

Melt marshmallows in saucepan with reserved pineapple juice, stirring constantly. Let cool slightly. Add gradually to cream cheese, beating until thoroughly blended. Add pineapple tidbits and fruit cocktail. Refrigerate until set.

Grapefruit Salad

1 (3–ounce) package lemon
   gelatin
¾ cup boiling water
1 cup grapefruit juice

¼ teaspoon salt
1 tablespoon sugar
2 cups grapefruit sections
½ tablespoon onion, grated

Dissolve gelatin in boiling water. Add grapefruit juice. Add seasonings and chill. When beginning to thicken, fold in grapefruit and onions. Mold and serve.

Heavenly Hash

1 (#2) can fruit cocktail,
   drained
1 (#2) can pineapple chunks,
   drained
1 (6–ounce) jar maraschino
   cherries, drained

1 (8–ounce) carton fat–free sour
   cream
3 cups miniature
   marshmallows
⅛ teaspoon coconut extract

Combine drained fruits and cherries. In a separate bowl, combine sour cream, marshmallows and extract; mixing well. Add fruit and cherries, tossing well. Refrigerate several hours before serving.

Holiday Cranberry Salad

2 (3–ounce) packages
   strawberry gelatin
2 cups boiling water
2 cups sugar

1 package fresh cranberries
1 orange, peeled and seeded
1 apple, peeled and cored

Dissolve gelatin with water and sugar. Coarsely grind fruits and add to the mixture. Refrigerate until set.

Hot Fruit Salad

1 (#2) can sliced peaches	⅓ cup Fleischmann's Fat Free
1 (#2) can sliced pears	Squeezable Spread
1 (#2) can chunk pineapple	¾ cup brown sugar
1 (#2) can black cherries	1 (#2) can applesauce
1 cup fresh strawberries	3 tablespoons brown sugar
2 large bananas	

Drain fruit well. Bring Fleischmann's, brown sugar and applesauce to boil. Pour over fruit and refrigerate overnight. Next day add sliced bananas and pour into a Pam–sprayed 2 quart baking dish. Bake at 350° for 45 minutes. Remove from oven and sprinkle with 3 tablespoons brown sugar. Return to oven for 10 to 15 minutes.

Honeydew Ring with Fruit

1 honeydew melon	Orange juice

Cut rings of a honeydew melon about 1–inch thick. Remove all seeds; peel rind. Fill hole with fruits, any kind, such as peaches, apricots, white grapes, black cherries, red plums, strawberries, pineapples, bananas, etc. Pour orange juice over fruit and ring. Sift confectioners sugar over all. Place in refrigerator. Sugar will crystallize. Serve chilled.

Lemon–Ginger Oranges

½ cup orange juice	½ teaspoon grated orange peel
¼ cup fresh lemon juice	½ teaspoon powdered ginger
¼ cup honey	3 cups fresh orange slices
½ teaspoon grated lemon peel	

Combine first 6 ingredients in saucepan. Bring to a boil. Simmer for 5 minutes. Pour over oranges. Let chill for at least 4 hours before serving.

Hot Spiced Fruit I

1 (6–ounce) jar maraschino
    cherries, drained
1 (16–ounce) can apricots in
    light syrup
1 (16–ounce) can peaches in
    light syrup
1 (16–ounce) can pears in light
    syrup

1 (8–ounce) can pineapple
    chunks
⅓ cup orange juice
2 tablespoons brown sugar
2 teaspoons orange rind,
    freshly grated
4 ounces chopped dates

Drain fruit, reserving liquid from each fruit except for cherries. Combine juices with orange juice, brown sugar and rind in saucepan. Bring to a boil and simmer, uncovered, until liquid is reduced to almost half, about 10 to 15 minutes. Meanwhile, cut fruit into bite–sized pieces. Add fruit to hot liquid and heat through. Serve immediately.

Hot Spiced Fruit II

1 pound canned peach halves
1 pound canned pear halves
1 pound canned pineapple
    chunks
1 (6–ounce) jar maraschino
    cherries, halved

½ cup orange marmalade
2 tablespoons Ultra Promise
    70% Less Fat
1 stick cinnamon
½ teaspoon nutmeg
½ teaspoon ground cloves

Drain fruit well reserving 1½ cups syrup; add to syrup, marmalade, Promise, cinnamon, nutmeg and cloves. Bring to boil and cook 3 minutes. Reduce heat. Gently stir in fruit. Heat thoroughly, approximately 20 minutes.

Lemon–Lime Mold

1 (3–ounce) package lemon
  gelatin
1 (3–ounce) package lime
  gelatin
24 large marshmallows,
  quartered

3 cups boiling water
6 ounces fat–free cream cheese
2 tablespoons vinegar
1 (#2) can crushed pineapple

Pour boiling water over gelatin and marshmallows. Stir until marshmallows are melted and gelatin is dissolved. Chill. Blend cream
cheese with vinegar until smooth. Add pineapple juice, blending
thoroughly. Add pineapple and mix. Chill. When mixture is ready to
thicken, combine the two mixtures and mold as desired.

Lettuce and Fruit Salad

Lettuce, washed
Strawberries, washed, capped
  and halved

Grapefruit sections
Poppy Seed Dressing
  (see page 67)

Make a bed of lettuce on salad dish. Top with strawberries and
grapefruit. Drizzle dressing over top.

Luncheon Salad

1 (3–ounce) package lemon
  gelatin
1 (#2) can crushed pineapple,
  drained and juice reserved
6 ounces fat–free cream cheese

1 (2–ounce) jar pimentos
1 cup celery, finely chopped
1 cup evaporated skimmed
  milk, whipped

Heat gelatin in pineapple juice. Allow to cool. Gradually add cream
cheese, beating well after each addition. Add pimento and celery.
Fold in whipped milk. Refrigerate overnight. Serve on lettuce bed.

Mandarin Orange and Wild Rice Salad

1½ cups wild rice
4½ cups boiling water
3 green onions, sliced
1 small red onion, thinly sliced
1 (11–ounce) can mandarin
    oranges, drained

1 tablespoon orange rind,
    freshly grated
Salt and pepper to taste
Italian Vinaigrette Dressing
    (see page 75)

Bring water to a boil; add rice; cover and simmer over low heat until rice is cracked and puffy, about 50 to 55 minutes. Drain rice and chill. Add onions, oranges, orange rind, salt and pepper. Add Vinaigrette Dressing and toss gently. Refrigerate.

Mrs. Proctor's Orange Jello Salad

1 (3–ounce) package orange
    gelatin
1 (3–ounce) package lemon
    gelatin
2 cups boiling water
1 large can crushed pineapple
    with juice

2 small cans mandarin oranges,
    drained
½ cup Weight Watcher's Fat
    Free Whipped Dressing
½ cup marshmallows
1 cup Dream Whip, prepared
    (see page 329), or Cool Whip
    Free

Dissolve gelatins in boiling water. Add pineapple with juice and mandarin oranges. Congeal until firm. Combine whipped dressing and marshmallows. Fold in Dream Whip or Cool Whip Free. Spread over gelatin.

Orange Salad

1 (16–ounce) carton fat–free
    cottage cheese, drained
1 (3–ounce) package orange
    gelatin
1 (11–ounce) can mandarin
    oranges, drained

1 (20–ounce) can crushed
    pineapple, drained
2 envelopes Dream Whip,
    prepared (see page 329), or
    Cool Whip Free

Sprinkle gelatin over cottage cheese and stir. Add drained fruit. Fold in Dream Whip or Cool Whip Free and chill.

Orange–Pineapple Salad

1 (3–ounce) box orange jello
1 pint fat–free cottage cheese
1 (11–ounce) can mandarin
  oranges, drained

2 cups Dream Whip, prepared
  (see page 329), or Cool Whip
  Free
1 (16–ounce) can crushed
  pineapple, drained

Mix together all ingredients except for Dream Whip or Cool Whip Free, mixing thoroughly. Fold in Dream Whip or Cool Whip Free. Chill.

Peach Brandy Salad

1 (3–ounce) package lemon
  gelatin
1 cup boiling water
⅔ cup cold water

1 (#2) can peaches, chopped,
  drained and reserving ⅓ cup
  juice
½ cup celery, chopped fine
3 tablespoons brandy

Dissolve gelatin in boiling water. Add the ⅓ cup reserved peach juice and cold water. Refrigerate until slightly thickened. Stir in remaining ingredients. Chill until firm.

Peachy Salad

1 (16–ounce) can peaches,
  chopped, juice reserved
1 (3–ounce) package strawberry
  gelatin

1 (8–ounce) package fat–free
  cream cheese
1 cup Dream Whip, prepared
  (see page 329), or Cool Whip
  Free

Add water to reserved juice to make 1¼ cups. Boil and add gelatin. Stir until dissolved. Blend together cream cheese and peaches in blender until well blended. Add gelatin to cream cheese mixture and process well. Remove from blender and whisk in Dream Whip or Cool Whip Free. Refrigerate until set.

Pear Salad I

1 (16–ounce) can pears, diced
  and juice reserved
1 (3–ounce) package lime
  gelatin

1 (8–ounce) package fat–free
  cream cheese
1 cup Dream Whip, prepared
  (see page 329), or Cool Whip
  Free

Add water to reserved juice to make 1¼ cups liquid. Boil and add gelatin, stirring until dissolved. Blend together cream cheese and pears in blender until well blended. Add gelatin to cream cheese mixture and process well. Remove from blender and whisk in Dream Whip or Cool Whip Free. Refrigerate until set.

Pear Salad II

Fresh pears
Romaine lettuce, washed and
  chopped

Fat–free blue cheese dressing

Wash and core pears; slice thinly. Add lettuce and toss with blue cheese dressing.

Raspberry Salad

1 (3–ounce) package raspberry
  gelatin
1 (8–ounce) package fat–free
  cream cheese
¼ cup Weight Watcher's Fat
  Free Whipped Dressing

1 banana, sliced
1 (11–ounce) can crushed
  pineapple
½ cup Dream Whip, prepared
  (see page 329), or Cool Whip
  Free

Dissolve gelatin in 1 cup boiling water. Set aside to cool. Mix together cream cheese and whipped dressing and add to cooled gelatin; stir until smooth. Add remaining ingredients. Chill until firm.

Red Raspberry Delight

2 (10–ounce) packages frozen
   raspberries, thawed
2 (3–ounce) packages red
   raspberry gelatin

2 cups boiling water
1 (16–ounce) can applesauce
2 tablespoons sugar

Drain raspberries reserving 1 cup juice. Dissolve gelatin in boiling water; stir in reserved juice, applesauce and sugar. Chill until partially set. Fold in raspberries. Pour into a 6–cup mold ring. Chill until firm.

Spicy Fruit Salad

1 jar spiced peaches, diced and
   liquid reserved
2 (3–ounce) packages lemon
   gelatin
¾ cup water

4 large oranges, peeled,
   sectioned and cut
1 (6–ounce) jar maraschino
   cherries, drained and diced

Drain peaches and heat juice with water. Dissolve gelatin with juice mixture. Cool gelatin mixture and add fruits. Pour into mold and refrigerate until set.

24–Hour Fruit Salad

⅓ cup fresh lemon juice
1 teaspoon lemon rind, grated
⅓ cup pineapple juice
¼ cup sugar
2 tablespoons flour
¼ teaspoon salt
1 Egg Beater
1 cup pineapple, diced

1 (#2) can seeded white cherries
1 small can mandarin oranges,
   drained
1 cup marshmallows
¾ cup Dream Whip, prepared
   (see page 329), or Cool Whip
   Free

Blend lemon juice, lemon rind, pineapple juice, sugar, flour, salt and Egg Beater in saucepan; cook until thickened, stirring frequently. Cool. Fold Dream Whip or Cool Whip Free into cooled juice mixture. Combine fruits and marshmallows; add to creamed mixture. Refrigerate for at least 24 hours before serving.

White Wine Fruit

2 tablespoons sugar
½ cup dry white wine
2 tablespoons fresh lemon
juice

4 cups honeydew balls
4 cups cantaloupe balls
1 cup seedless white grapes

In a mixing bowl combine sugar, wine and lemon juice, stirring until sugar has dissolved. Add fruit. Gently toss. Refrigerate for at least 2 hours, tossing occasionally. Drain and serve on bed of lettuce.

White Wine Fruit Salad

1 (16–ounce) can pear halves,
undrained
⅓ cup golden raisins

½ cup dried apricot halves
¼ cup white wine
1 teaspoon sugar

Combine fruit and wine; toss gently coating fruit well. Chill for several hours before serving.

Wild Rice and Blueberry Salad

⅔ cup wild rice
1½ cups water
Salt to taste
½ cup dried blueberries, cut in
half
¼ cup purple onions, finely
chopped

3 tablespoons celery, finely
chopped
1 teaspoon fresh lime rind,
grated
2 tablespoons cider vinegar
Pinch of sugar

Combine rice, water and salt and cook as directed on package. Rinse under cold running water and drain well. While rice is cooking, prepare vegetables and blueberries. Toss with vinegar and sugar. Be careful not to oversweeten with the sugar. It will take away from the natural sweetness of the blueberries.

Wild Rice and Cranberry Salad

⅔ cup wild rice
1½ cups water
Salt to taste
½ cup dried cranberries, cut in
  half
¼ cup purple onions, finely
  diced

3 tablespoons celery, finely
  diced
1 teaspoon fresh orange rind,
  shredded
2 tablespoons cider vinegar
Pinch of sugar

Combine rice, water and salt and cook as directed on package. Rinse under cold running water and drain well. While rice is cooking, prepare vegetables and cranberries. Toss with vinegar and sugar. Be careful not to oversweeten with the sugar. It will take away from the natural sweetness of the cranberries.

Winter Fruit Compote

1 cup sliced apples (canned)
1 cup pears, sliced
1 cup cranberries, whole
1 cup dried apricots, halved
½ cup white raisins

1 (22–ounce) can lemon pie
  filling
¼ cup Grand Marnier
1 teaspoon cinnamon
¼ teaspoon nutmeg

Layer fruits in order listed in a Pam–sprayed 9 x 13–inch casserole dish. Mix remaining ingredients and pour over fruit. Bake, covered, at 350° for 1 hour. Let sit for 45 minutes before serving.

Crabmeat Salad

1 cup imitation crabmeat
2 (#2) cans artichoke hearts,
  chopped
2 egg whites, boiled and diced
¼ cup mushrooms, thinly
  sliced

¼ cup Weight Watcher's Fat
  Free Whipped Dressing
2 tablespoons vinegar
1 tablespoon chives, snipped
Salt and pepper to taste

Combine all ingredients. Refrigerate for several hours so that flavors can blend. Serve on lettuce leaf with lemon wedges.

Chicken Cranberry Layer Salad

1ST LAYER:

2 envelopes unflavored gelatin
½ cup cold water
1 cup Weight Watcher's Fat
 Free Whipped Dressing
1 teaspoon salt
3 tablespoons lemon juice

1 cup celery, finely chopped
2 tablespoons parsley flakes
1 tablespoon chives
2 cups chicken breasts, cooked
 and finely chopped

Dissolve gelatin in water. Heat on low. Add to remaining ingredients. Pour into a 9 x 13–inch Pam–sprayed dish. Chill until firm.

2ND LAYER:

1 envelope unflavored gelatin
1 (16–ounce) can whole
 cranberry sauce

1 (9–ounce) can crushed
 pineapple, drained

Mix all ingredients and pour over chicken. Chill until firm.

Chicken Oriental Salad

½ teaspoon sugar
¼ cup teriyaki sauce
¼ cup dry sherry
2 tablespoons vinegar
2 tablespoons water
2 cups chicken breasts, boned,
 cooked and cut into thin
 strips

½ cup celery, bias–sliced
½ cup water chestnuts, sliced
2 tablespoons green onion,
 sliced
1 medium cantaloupe, balls or
 cubed
Lettuce

Combine first 5 ingredients and mix well. In a bowl combine chicken, celery, chestnuts and onions. Pour marinade over; toss to coat. Cover and refrigerate 2 to 3 hours. To serve, place on lettuce bed or in lettuce cups; add cantaloupe to chicken mixture. Lift salad from marinade with slotted spoon; spoon each serving onto lettuce bed or into lettuce cup.

Chicken Curry Salad

4 chicken breasts, cooked and
  diced
1 cup celery, finely chopped
1 apple, pared and chopped
¼ cup green pepper, chopped

½ cup Weight Watcher's Fat
  Free Whipped Dressing
½ cup fat–free sour cream
½ teaspoon curry powder
Salt and pepper to taste

Mix together whipped dressing, sour cream and curry. Add remaining ingredients. Refrigerate for several hours allowing flavors to blend.

Chicken Pasta Salad

12 ounces rainbow rotini
3 chicken bouillon cubes
4 cups broccoli flowerets
1 cup chicken breasts, skinned,
  cooked and chopped

2 cups Weight Watcher's Fat
  Free Whipped Dressing
Salt and pepper to taste

Cook pasta according to directions but adding chicken bouillon to water. Drain and cool pasta. Add remaining ingredients and chill.

Chicken Salad

1 cup chicken, cooked and
  finely diced
2 egg whites, boiled and diced
3 heaping tablespoons Weight
  Watcher's Fat Free Whipped
  Dressing

1 tablespoon sweet pickle
  relish
1 tablespoon onion, extra
  finely chopped
Salt and pepper to taste

Mix all ingredients; stir well. Keep refrigerated.

Chicken Salad Surprise

1 (3–ounce) package lemon
  gelatin
1 cup boiling water
1 cup chicken breasts, cooked
  and diced

1 cup Weight Watcher's Fat
  Free Whipped Dressing
1 cup green seedless grapes,
  sliced
¼ cup celery, finely chopped

Dissolve gelatin in the boiling water. Add remaining ingredients. Refrigerate until set.

Chicken Waldorf Salad

2 cups cooked chicken breast,
  cubed
½ cup apple, chopped
½ cup celery, chopped

2 tablespoons raisins
½ cup Weight Watcher's Fat
  Free Whipped Dressing

Mix all ingredients until well blended. Serve on lettuce leaves.

Cold Pasta & Chicken

½ pound vermicelli
1 tablespoon fat–free
  vinaigrette salad dressing
1½ cups Herb Majic Fat Free
  sweet 'n sour salad dressing
1 cup broccoli flowerets,
  blanched

1 cup green peas, cooked and
  drained
2 cups chicken, cooked and
  chopped
⅓ cup chopped fresh basil
Cherry tomatoes

Cook pasta according to package directions. Mix together the salad dressings. Using ½ cup dressing, toss with pasta. Cool and chill at least 3 hours. In separate bowl, toss vegetables with remaining dressing. Cover and chill. When ready to serve, add chicken to pasta and toss. Add vegetables and basil.

Crab Louis

1 head lettuce
12 ounces fresh, canned or
  imitation crabmeat
3 egg whites, hard–boiled and
  cut into wedges
2 large tomatoes, cut into
  wedges
1 cup Weight Watcher's Fat
  Free Whipped Dressing

¼ cup fat–free sour cream
¼ cup chili sauce
¼ cup onions, finely chopped
1 teaspoon lemon juice
1 teaspoon parsley flakes
Salt and pepper to taste
Paprika (optional)

Put each salad together individually. Layer lettuce then crabmeat and top with tomatoes and egg whites. In a separate bowl, combine remaining ingredients to make dressing. Pour dressing over salad. May be sprinkled with paprika.

Crab Salad

1½ cups imitation crabmeat,
  processed finely chopped
¼ cup Weight Watcher's Fat
  Free Whipped Dressing

1 teaspoon lemon juice
½ teaspoon horseradish

Combine all ingredients. Let set in refrigerator for several hours to let flavors blend.

Crunchy Chicken Salad

½ cup Weight Watcher's Fat
  Free Whipped Dressing
2 tablespoons skim milk
1 tablespoon cider vinegar
2 teaspoons onion, grated
1 teaspoon salt

2 cups chicken breasts, cooked
  and diced
1 large green pear, cubed
1 large red apple, cubed
1 cup celery, thinly sliced
¼ cup green pepper, chopped

In a large bowl add first 5 ingredients. Add remaining ingredients. Toss gently until well mixed.

Fruit and Chicken Salad

2 cups chicken breasts, skinned, cooked, boned and diced
3 cups rice, cooked
1 cup celery, finely sliced
¼ cup green pepper, chopped
1 (13.25–ounce) can pineapple tidbits, drained
½ cup seedless grapes, halved
2 tablespoons pimento, sliced
¼ cup fat–free sour cream
½ cup Weight Watcher's Fat Free Whipped Dressing
2 teaspoons salt
1 teaspoon curry powder

Combine chicken, rice, celery, pepper, pineapple, grapes and pimento. In separate bowl, blend remaining ingredients. Toss lightly. Chill. May be served on a bed of lettuce.

Healthy Ham Salad

3 cups Healthy Choice ham, finely chopped
1½ cups fat–free Cheddar cheese, shredded
2 cups apples, peeled and diced
1 cup celery, finely chopped
¾ cup Weight Watcher's Fat Free Whipped Dressing

Combine all ingredients and mix well. Refrigerate several hours so that flavors can blend.

Niçoise Salad

4 medium new potatoes, cut into fourths
1 (10–ounce) package frozen whole green beans, thawed
6 cups Bibb lettuce, torn into bite–size pieces
2 cups chicken breasts, cooked and diced
2 egg whites, hard–boiled and cut into wedges
Dijon Basil Vinaigrette (see page 66)

Place potatoes and enough water to cover in a medium saucepan. Cook over medium heat for 10 minutes. Add green beans and continue cooking for another 10 minutes. Drain. Cover and refrigerate until chilled. Arrange lettuce on a serving platter. Top with chicken. Arrange potatoes, beans, tomatoes and eggs over chicken. Drizzle with Vinaigrette.

Orange Chicken Salad

2 cups cooked rice
½ cup celery, finely chopped
¼ cup onions, finely chopped
¼ cup green peppers, finely
  chopped
¼ cup water chestnuts, finely
  chopped

Mandarin orange sections
1¼ cups chicken breasts,
  cooked and chopped
½ cup fat–free Catalina
  dressing
1 tablespoon soy sauce
¼ teaspoon ginger

In bowl combine vegetables and chicken. In separate bowl combine Catalina, soy sauce and ginger. Toss with rice mixture. Garnish with mandarin oranges. Let chill several hours so that flavors can blend.

Shrimp & Grapefruit Pasta

1 (26–ounce) jar grapefruit
  sections
1 (16–ounce) package tri–color
  rotelle pasta
1 pound shrimp, peeled,
  deveined, cooked and
  drained
3 scallions, thinly sliced

1 red pepper, chopped
1 medium cucumber, diced
1 teaspoon dried celery seed
2 tablespoons cilantro,
  chopped
5 tablespoons rice wine vinegar
Black pepper to taste
¼ cup water

Drain grapefruit sections reserving ¼ cup of liquid. In a small bowl, place reserved liquid, vinegar, pepper and water. Set aside. In a large bowl combine drained grapefruit and next 7 ingredients. Pour vinegar mixture over pasta mixture and toss gently. Serve chilled.

Shrimp and Macaroni Salad

8 ounces macaroni, cooked
6 egg whites, hard boiled and diced
½ cup celery, finely chopped
1 cup carrots, grated

1½ pounds shrimp, cooked, peeled, and deveined, without tails, and chilled
Salt and pepper to taste
Weight Watcher's Fat Free Whipped Dressing

Mix all ingredients adding enough dressing to hold together. Refrigerate for several hours so that flavors can blend.

Taco Salad

¾ pound ground round
1 package taco seasoning mix
1 medium head lettuce, shredded
½ green pepper, chopped
3 ribs celery, chopped

2 tomatoes, peeled and chopped
1 cup fat–free Cheddar cheese, shredded
Salt and pepper to taste
Low–fat baked tortilla chips

Cook ground round in a colander in microwave until done. Place in skillet. Add taco seasoning, tossing well. Add all other ingredients excluding tortilla chips. Heat thoroughly. Serve with tortilla chips and/or picante sauce.

Tuna Salad

2 (7–ounce) cans white tuna
1 cup pineapple chunks,
    drained
3 cups carrots, grated

1 cup celery, finely chopped
1 cup raisins
1 cup Weight Watcher's Fat
    Free Whipped Dressing
Salt and white pepper to taste

Mix all ingredients well. Serve on bed of lettuce.

Tuna–Stuffed Tomatoes

1 can spring water tuna,
    drained
4 tablespoons Weight
    Watcher's Fat Free Whipped
    Dressing
2 eggs, boiled, diced and yolks
    discarded

1 tablespoon sweet pickle
    relish
1 tablespoon onion, finely
    diced
1 tablespoon parsley flakes
Salt and pepper to taste
4 medium tomatoes

Wash and core tomatoes; set aside. In a small bowl, mix remaining ingredients. Dip ¼ of the tuna mixture in each tomato.

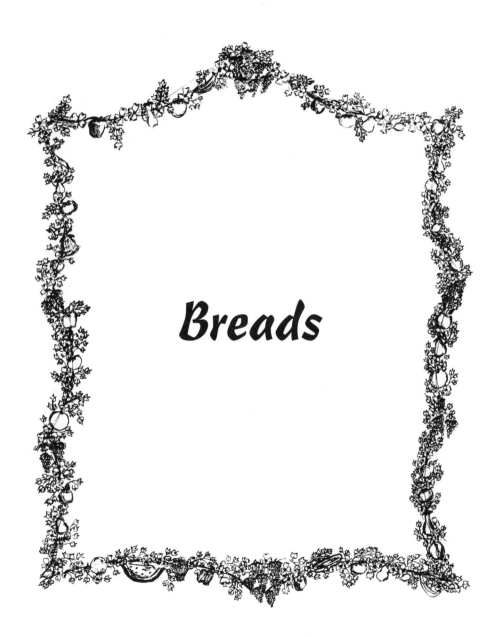

Breads

Basic Bread

1 package dry yeast
½ cup warm water
3 teaspoons sugar

4 cups self–rising flour
1½ cups water

Dissolve yeast and sugar in warm water. Add flour, water and yeast mixture. Knead well. Let rise until double in bulk. Punch down and knead briefly. Divide dough and place in Pam–sprayed loaf pans. Bake at 375° for 35 minutes or until done.

Batter Bread

3½ cups self–rising flour
½ cup dry non–fat powdered
  milk
1 teaspoon salt
1 cup quick oats
1 tablespoon sugar

1½ cups water, divided
1 package dry yeast
2 Egg Beaters
¼ cup Ultra Promise 70% Less
  Fat

Mix dry ingredients. Cut in Ultra Promise. Dissolve yeast in ¼ cup warm water. Add remaining water and Egg Beaters to yeast mixture. Add to dry ingredients and mix well. Place dough in two Pam–sprayed loaf pans. Let rise 1 hour. Bake at 350° for 30 minutes or until done.

Sally Lunn Bread

1 package dry yeast
1 tablespoon water
2 cups lukewarm skim milk
¼ cup Ultra Promise 70% Less
  Fat

4 cups self–rising flour
2 Egg Beaters
1 teaspoon salt
Butter salt

In a mixing bowl, dissolve yeast and sugar in the lukewarm milk. Stir in Promise. Mix flour into the mixture and stir well. Add Egg Beaters and salt; beat until smooth. Pour batter into 2 Pam–sprayed 9 x 5–inch loaf pans or 1 Pam–sprayed 8 x 12–inch loaf pan. Cover with cloth and let rise in a warm place until doubled in bulk (about 1½ hours). Bake in 375° oven for 30 minutes.

Braided Onion Bread

1 package dry yeast
¼ cup warm water
4 cups self–rising flour
¼ cup sugar
1½ teaspoons salt
½ cup hot water

½ cup skim milk
⅛ cup Ultra Promise 70% Less Fat
⅛ cup Fleischmann's Fat Free Squeezable Spread
1 Egg Beater

FILLING:
¼ cup Ultra Promise 70% Less Fat
⅛ cup Butter Buds Liquid (see page 50)
1 tablespoon fat–free Parmesan cheese

1 tablespoon poppy seed or sesame seeds
1 teaspoon garlic salt
1 teaspoon paprika

Dissolve yeast in warm water. Add 2 cups flour and remaining ingredients. Beat 2 minutes at medium speed.

Stir in remaining flour by hand. Put dough in a Pam–sprayed bowl; cover and let rise approximately 1 hour or until doubled in bulk.

Combine all filling ingredients and set aside.

Punch dough down. Knead on floured surface until dough is not sticky. Roll out to an 18 x 12–inch rectangle. Spread filling over dough.

Cut rectangle into three 18 x 4–inch strips. On a Pam–sprayed cookie sheet, braid strips. Cover and let rise for 1 hour.

Bake at 350° for 30 to 35 minutes. DO NOT OVERBAKE.

Cinnamon Swirl Bread

1 package yeast
¼ cup warm water
2 cups skim milk, scalded
⅓ cup sugar

2 teaspoons salt
¼ cup Ultra Promise 70% Less
   Fat
6 cups self–rising flour

CINNAMON MIXTURE:
½ cup sugar
1 tablespoon cinnamon

3 teaspoons water

Dissolve yeast in warm water. Combine milk, sugar, salt and Promise; cool to lukewarm. Stir in 2 cups flour; mix well. Add yeast mixture; mix. Add remaining flour. Knead until smooth. Place in a Pam–sprayed bowl. Cover. Let rise in warm place for 1 hour and 15 minutes. Punch down. Roll dough into two 15 x 7–inch rectangles. Sprinkle each with 1½ teaspoons water. Sprinkle with half of the cinnamon mixture. Roll into loaves and place in 2 Pam–sprayed 9 x 5 x 3–inch loaf pans. Cover and let rise 45 minutes. Bake at 350° for 20 minutes or until done.

GLAZE:
1 cup 10X sugar
1 tablespoon Ultra Promise
   70% Less Fat

⅛ teaspoon vanilla
1½ tablespoons skim milk

Mix first 3 ingredients. Use enough milk to make a thick glaze. Brush on bread while bread is warm.

Dill Bread

1 package active dry yeast	2 teaspoons dill weed
¾ cup warm water	2 tablespoons minced dried
1 cup small curd fat–free	onion
cottage cheese, room	½ teaspoon salt
temperature	1 Egg Beater
2 tablespoons sugar	2½ to 2¾ cups self–rising flour

Soften yeast in water; set aside. In large bowl, mix next 6 ingredients. Add this to the yeast mixture. Gradually add flour, stirring after each addition, until has a smooth, non–sticky texture. Knead dough. DO NOT OVER KNEAD.

Place dough in a Pam–sprayed bowl; cover and set in a warm place and let rise until doubled in bulk, about 1¼ hours. Punch dough and lightly knead. Place in a Pam–sprayed 9 x 5 x 3–inch loaf pan. Let rise about 45 minutes. Lightly spray top of bread with butter flavored Pam spray. Bake at 350° for 35 to 38 minutes.

Pepper Cheese Bread

1 package yeast	1 cup fat–free sour cream
¼ cup hot water	1 cup fat–free mozzarella
2½ cups self–rising flour	cheese, shredded
1 Egg Beater	½ teaspoon coarse black
2 tablespoons sugar	pepper

In a large mixing bowl, dissolve yeast in hot water. Add half of the flour, Egg Beater, sugar and sour cream. Mix with mixer on low speed for 30 seconds, then on high speed for 2 minutes. With a spoon, stir in remaining flour, cheese and pepper. Place in a Pam–sprayed 9 x 5 x 3–inch loaf pan. Bake at 350° for 30 minutes. Aluminum foil may be placed over bread the last 10 minutes to prevent over browning.

Potato Bread

1½ cups water
1 medium potato, peeled and
   diced
1 cup non–fat buttermilk
3 tablespoons sugar

2 tablespoons Ultra Promise
   70% Less Fat
6 to 6½ cups self–rising flour
2 packages dry yeast

In a saucepan, combine water and potato. Bring to boiling. Cook, uncovered, until very tender. DO NOT DRAIN. Mash potato in water. Measure potato mixture. If necessary, add additional water to make 1¾ cups total. Return mixture to saucepan. Add buttermilk, sugar, and Promise. Heat or cool as necessary to 120° to 130°. In a large bowl combine 2 cups of flour and yeast. Add potato mixture. With an electric mixer on medium speed, beat for 30 seconds, scraping bowl. Then beat on high for 3 minutes. Using a spoon, stir in as much of the remaining flour as you can.

On a lightly floured surface, knead in enough remaining flour to make a moderately stiff dough that is smooth (about 6 to 8 minutes). Shape into a ball. Place in a Pam–sprayed bowl. Cover and let rise in a warm place until doubled (45 to 60 minutes).

Punch down. Turn out onto a lightly floured surface. Divide in half. Place in Pam–sprayed 8 x 4 x 2–inch loaf pans. Cover and let rise until nearly double (about 30 minutes).

Bake at 375° for 25 to 30 minutes or until done. Cover with foil the last 15 minutes of baking to prevent over browning.

Richard and Ariadna's Russian Black Bread

3 to 4 cups bread flour
2 cups All–Bran cereal
2 packages active dry yeast
1 tablespoon sugar
1 tablespoon instant coffee
1 tablespoon salt
2 teaspoons onion powder

2½ cups water
½ cup molasses
¼ cup Ultra Promise 70% Less Fat
3 tablespoons cocoa
3 cups medium rye flour

Pam–spray two 8–inch or 9–inch round cake pans. In a large bowl, combine 2½ cups bread flour, cereal, yeast, sugar, coffee, salt, and onion powder. In large saucepan, heat water, molasses, Promise, and cocoa until very warm (120° to 130°). Add warm liquid to flour mixture. Blend at low speed until moistened. Beat 3 minutes at medium speed.

By hand, stir in rye flour plus enough bread flour to form a stiff dough. Knead on floured surface adding ½ to 1 cup bread flour until dough is smooth and elastic, about 10 minutes. (Dough will be slightly sticky). Place in a Pam–sprayed bowl, cover loosely with plastic wrap and top with a cloth towel. Let rise in a warm place until doubled in size, 1 to 1½ hours.

Punch down dough. Let rest on counter with inverted bowl for about 15 minutes. Divide dough in half. Place in pie plates and shape into round loaves. If desired, brush tops with mixture of 1 egg white and 1 tablespoon water. Bake at 375° for 40 to 50 minutes until crust is dark brown and loaves sound hollow when lightly tapped. Remove from pans immediately.

Savory Cheese Bread

1 loaf French bread, sliced to
  bottom crust
1 tablespoon mustard
3 tablespoons Ultra Promise
  70% Less Fat
¼ cup Butter Buds Liquid
  (see page 50)

¼ cup minced onion
1 tablespoon poppy seed
Fat–free Swiss cheese slices
I Can't Believe It's Not Butter
  spray

Mix together mustard, Promise, Butter Buds, onion and poppy seed. Spread mustard mixture between bread slices. Add cheese slices between bread slices. Wrap in foil. Leave top uncovered. Bake at 400° for 15 minutes. Spray top with Butter Spray before serving.

Whole Wheat Pita Bread

2 tablespoons sugar
2 cups water
4 cups all–purpose flour

2 cups whole wheat flour
1 package dry yeast
1 teaspoon salt

Preheat oven to 500°. Dissolve sugar in water and set aside. Combine 2 cups flour, yeast and salt in a large bowl. Add water mixture and blend well. Gradually add remaining 4 cups flour, mixing thoroughly. Cover and let rise 20 minutes. Knead in bowl. Divide dough into eighths. Roll each one into large circles. Place on ungreased cookie sheet. Let rise in a warm, draft free place for 3 minutes. Bake on middle rack for 6 to 8 minutes or until a pale beige color. Cool. Cut in half and split carefully.

NOTE: Six cups all–purpose flour may be used instead of mixing with wheat flour.

Cinnamon–Raisin Biscuits

1 cup self–rising flour
¼ cup sugar
1 teaspoon cinnamon

2 tablespoons Weight
  Watcher's Fat Free Whipped
  Dressing
¼ cup skim milk

Mix together dry ingredients. Add whipped dressing and mix until mixture resembles cornmeal. Add milk; mix until flour lets go of bowl. Turn on a floured surface and lightly knead. Roll and cut into biscuits. Bake at 425° for 10 to 12 minutes or until done. Makes 10 biscuits.

GLAZE:
½ tablespoon Ultra Promise
  70% Less Fat

¼ cup 10X sugar
½ teaspoon skim milk

Blend Promise and sugar together. Add milk and blend well. Ice biscuits while warm.

Potato Biscuits

½ cup sugar
2 packages dry yeast
1 tablespoon salt
1½ cups warm water
¼ cup Butter Buds Liquid
  (see page 50)

¼ cup Ultra Promise 70% Less
  Fat
½ cup Egg Beaters
½ cup potatoes, cooked,
  unseasoned, cooled and
  mashed
6½ cups self–rising flour

In a small mixing bowl, combine first 4 ingredients. In a large mixing bowl, combine next 4 ingredients. Add yeast mixture to potato mixture. Add flour gradually. Mix until dough turns loose of bowl. Transfer dough to a Pam–sprayed bowl, cover and let set in a warm place to rise. After dough has doubled, punch down. You may roll out as much dough as desired. Cut with a biscuit cutter. Let rise 1½ to 2 hours in a warm place. Bake at 400° for 30 minutes. Place remaining dough in refrigerator. Will keep 2 or 3 days, but punch down daily.

Cinnamon–Raisin Scones

1 teaspoon ground cinnamon
1 tablespoon sugar
1½ cups all–purpose flour
1½ teaspoons baking powder
½ teaspoon salt
¼ cup sugar
¼ cup Ultra Promise 70% Less
   Fat
¼ cup Fleischmann's Fat Free
   Squeezable Spread
½ cup raisins
¼ cup fat–free sour cream
¼ cup orange juice
2 teaspoons grated orange peel
Devonshire Clotted Cream
   (see page 329)

Mix together cinnamon and 1 tablespoon sugar and set aside.

In small mixing bowl, combine flour, baking powder, salt and sugar.
Cut in Promise. Add Fleischmann's, raisins, sour cream, orange juice
and peel; mix until well blended. Turn dough onto lightly floured
surface. Roll to ½–inch thickness. Place scones on a Pam–sprayed
baking sheet. Sprinkle with cinnamon and sugar mixture. Bake at
400° for 8 minutes.

Serve with strawberry preserves or preserves of your choice and
Devonshire Clotted Cream.

Lemon Poppy Seed Scones

1½ cups all–purpose flour
1½ teaspoons baking powder
½ teaspoon salt
¼ cup sugar
¼ cup Ultra Promise 70% Less
   Fat
¼ cup Fleischmann's Fat Free
   Squeezable Spread
1 teaspoon poppy seeds
¼ cup lemon juice
¼ cup fat–free sour cream
Devonshire Clotted Cream
   (see page 329)

In small mixing bowl, combine flour, baking powder, salt and sugar.
Cut in Promise. Add Fleischmann's, lemon juice, sour cream and
poppy seed, and mix until well blended. Turn dough onto lightly
floured surface. Knead lightly. Roll into ½–inch thickness. Place
scones on a Pam–sprayed baking sheet. Bake at 400° for 8 minutes.
Serve with preserves of your choice and Devonshire Clotted Cream.

Herb Biscuits

1 (10–count) tube canned
  biscuits (1 fat gram or less
  per biscuit)
½ teaspoon celery seeds
1 teaspoon dried parsley
½ teaspoon dill weed

2 tablespoons onion flakes
1 tablespoon fat–free Parmesan
  cheese
Pam Butter spray
I Can't Believe It's Not Butter
  spray

Combine dry seasonings. Spray biscuits with Pam Butter spray. Sprinkle ½ of the seasoning mixture on biscuits. Turn biscuits over. Spray with Pam Butter spray and sprinkle with remaining seasonings. Place in a Pam–sprayed loaf pan. Cook at 375° for 10 minutes. Spray with I Can't Believe It's Not Butter spray when done.

Baking Powder Biscuits

2½ cups all–purpose flour
½ teaspoon salt
3½ teaspoons baking powder
2 teaspoons sugar
¼ cup Ultra Promise 70% Less
  Fat

¾ cup skim milk
1 Egg Beater
1 egg white
1 tablespoon water

Sift together dry ingredients. Cut in Promise. Stir in milk and add egg. Roll into ¼–inch thickness. Brush tops with egg white and water mixture. Bake on Pam–sprayed baking pan at 375° for 15 minutes.

Mayonnaise Biscuits

1 cup self–rising flour
3 heaping tablespoons Weight
  Watcher's Fat Free Whipped
  Dressing

1 tablespoon sugar
½ cup skim milk
Scant salt

Mix flour, sugar and salt. Cut whipped dressing into dry mixture with a fork. Add milk; mix well. Drop by spoonfuls into Pam–sprayed muffin tin. Bake at 400° for 12 minutes.

Scones

1½ cups all–purpose flour	¼ cup Fleischmann's
1½ teaspoons baking powder	Squeezable Spread
½ teaspoon salt	¼ cup fat free sour cream
½ cup sugar	¼ cup skim milk
¼ cup Ultra Promise 70% Less Fat	Devonshire Clotted cream (see page 329)

In small bowl, combine flour, baking powder, salt and sugar. Cut in Promise. Add Fleischmann's, sour cream and milk. Mix until blended. Turn dough onto lightly floured surface. Knead lightly. Roll to ½–inch thickness. Place scones on a Pam–sprayed baking sheet. Bake at 400° for 8 minutes. Serve with preserves of your choice and Devonshire Clotted Cream.

Sweet Potato Biscuits

2 cups self–rising flour	6 tablespoons Ultra Promise
1 tablespoon baking powder	70% Less Fat
3 tablespoons sugar	¾ cup skim milk
¼ teaspoon nutmeg	1 cup mashed sweet potato, cooked

Mix together dry ingredients. Cut in Ultra Promise until it resembles the size of small peas. Stir milk into mashed potatoes. Gradually add to flour mixture, stirring from the center, until all dough is moistened. Turn out on floured surface and knead gently until dough comes together. Roll out to ½–inch thickness. Cut with a 2–inch biscuit cutter. Place on a Pam–sprayed cookie sheet. Bake at 425° for 8 minutes.

Bread Crumbs

1 loaf low–fat or fat–free bread

Trim crust from bread. Place on a baking sheet. Bake at 200° for 1 hour or until crunchy. Let cool and crumble. Store in an air tight container.

VARIATION: For seasoned bread crumbs, spray bread with Pam butter spray and sprinkle with Italian seasoning. Bake as directed, cool and crumble.

Italian Dijon Bread Sticks

1 envelope Italian dressing mix
¼ cup Dijon mustard
3 tablespoons Ultra Promise
   70% Less Fat

1 tablespoon fat–free Parmesan
   cheese
1 (11–ounce) package
   refrigerated soft bread sticks

Combine first 4 ingredients. Unroll dough. Cut in half crosswise and then cut each in half lengthwise. Separate strips and twist each slightly. Place on baking sheets. Generously brush with mustard mixture. Bake at 350° for 15 minutes or until lightly browned.

Garlic Croutons

1 teaspoon garlic powder
¾ teaspoon paprika
1 teaspoon dried parsley flakes
1 loaf sour dough French
   bread, cut into ½–inch cubes

Pam butter spray
I Can't Believe It's Not Butter
   spray

Spray cubed bread with Pam spray, tossing well so that bread is evenly coated. Add spices and continue tossing. Bake at 250° for 1 hour, stirring occasionally. Turn oven off but leave bread until bread is completely cooled. Lightly spray with I Can't Believe It's Not Butter spray.

Croutons

Wonder Light Low Fat bread   Pam butter spray
Italian seasoning, dried

Trim crust from bread. Cut bread into cubes. Spray bread with Pam spray, tossing until evenly coated. Sprinkle with Italian seasoning. Toss until well coated. Bake at 200° for 1 hour or until crunchy. Serve with soup or salads.

Crumpets

3 cups self–rising flour   ½ teaspoon soda
1½ teaspoons yeast   ½ teaspoon salt
1¾ cups warm water   ¾ cup skim milk, warmed

Blend flour, yeast and warm water together, cover with Pam–sprayed plastic and set aside to rise about 1 hour. Add soda and salt to warm milk and stir into the batter. Batter needs to be runny so you may have to add a little more milk. Cover again for 30 minutes to one hour. Heat non–stick skillet and spray with Pam. Spray muffin rings or tuna cans with both ends cut out. Place rings on griddle. Pour 2 tablespoons batter into each ring. Cook gently for 8 to 10 minutes or until well set and bubbles have burst. Remove rings, turn and continue cooking for 2 to 3 minutes.

Fritter Batter

1 cup self–rising flour   ⅓ cup non–fat buttermilk
2 teaspoons baking powder   1 tablespoon Ultra Promise
½ teaspoon salt   70% Less Fat
¼ cup sugar   Sugar
1 Egg Beater

Mix together dry ingredients. Add Egg Beater, milk and Ultra Promise. Stir lightly. Spoon into Pam–sprayed muffin tin. Bake at 350° for 7 minutes. While warm, roll into sugar.

Hush Puppies

2 cups self–rising cornmeal
1 cup self–rising flour
1½ teaspoons salt
2 Egg Beaters
¼ cup sugar

1½ cups skim milk
1 large onion, finely chopped
1 bell pepper, finely chopped
9 drops Tabasco

Combine dry ingredients. Add Egg Beaters and milk, stirring well. Add onion and bell pepper. Drop by spoonfuls into Pam–sprayed mini tins. Bake at 425° for 11 minutes. Makes approximately 5½ dozen.

Squash Fritters

2 cups yellow self–rising
  cornmeal
1 cup self–rising flour
1 cup squash
1 large onion

2 Egg Beaters
2 tablespoons sugar
¾ cup lowfat buttermilk
Salt to taste
Pepper to taste

Boil squash until tender. Put squash, onion and Egg Beaters in blender and liquefy; set aside. Mix in dry ingredients; add liquid from blender; add buttermilk. Let set 1 hour before cooking.

May be cooked in a Pam–sprayed non–stick moderately hot skillet until browned. Spray each patty with Pam before turning. Turn and cook an additional 2 minutes or until done.

OR

In a Pam–sprayed mini tin, drop mixture and bake at 425° for 6 minutes.

Mexican Cornbread

1½ cups self–rising yellow
cornmeal
1 cup cream style corn
¼ cup green pepper, finely
chopped
1 small onion, finely chopped
1 to 2 jalapeño peppers, extra
finely chopped

1 Egg Beater
1 cup fat–free Cheddar cheese,
shredded
3 tablespoons Ultra Promise
70% Less Fat, melted
¼ cup non–fat buttermilk

Mix together all ingredients. Pour into a Pam-sprayed baking dish. Bake at 400° for 35 minutes or until done. DO NOT OVER BAKE.

Whole Wheat Crust

1 cup whole–wheat self–rising
flour
2 tablespoons unbleached flour
½ cup Butter Buds Liquid
(see page 50)

2 tablespoons Ultra Promise
70% Less Fat
¼ teaspoon Mrs. Dash original
blend

Mix and chill. Roll out on lightly floured pastry sheet. Place on Pam-sprayed pie pan and trim edges. If recipe calls for baked crust, pierce bottom with a fork and bake at 350° until browned.

Carrot Bread

¼ cup Fleischmann's Fat Free
Squeezable Spread
3 tablespoons Ultra Promise
70% Less Fat
1 cup sugar

2 Egg Beaters
1½ cups self–rising flour
1 teaspoon cinnamon
1 cup carrots, grated

Cream together Fleischmann's, Promise and sugar. Mix Egg Beaters in well. Add flour and cinnamon and mix until smooth. Stir in carrots. Bake in a Pam–sprayed loaf pan. Bake at 350° for 28 minutes.

Apricot Bread with Glaze

1 (6–ounce) package dried
   apricots
1½ cups hot water
2 Egg Beaters

2 cups sugar
3½ cups self–rising flour
1 teaspoon salt
2 teaspoons vanilla extract

Combine apricots and water and set aside to cool. In a large mixing bowl, beat together Egg Beaters and sugar. Stir in fruit mixture. Add flour, salt and vanilla. Pour into Pam–sprayed loaf pan. Bake at 300° for 1 hour. After 15 minutes, cover top with aluminum foil to prevent over browning.

GLAZE:
¼ cup apricot nectar   ¼ cup sugar

Combine and stir until smooth. With knife, cut slits in warm bread. Pour glaze over all while hot.

Apricot Jam Bread

1½ cups self–rising flour
⅛ teaspoon salt
¼ cup sugar
1 Egg Beater
½ cup apricot jam

2 tablespoons Ultra Promise
   70% Less Fat
½ cup skim milk
Almond Glaze (see page 332)

Mix together dry ingredients; set aside. Beat Egg Beaters, jam, Promise and milk. Add to flour mixture and mix until moistened. Pour batter into Pam–sprayed loaf pan. Bake at 350° for 28 minutes.

Cherry Bread with Glaze

1 (6–ounce) jar maraschino
  cherries, cut into pieces
⅓ cup reserved cherry syrup
1½ cups self–rising flour

¼ teaspoon salt
2 Egg Beaters
¾ cup sugar

Mix together flour and salt. Beat Egg Beaters and sugar together. Alternately add dry ingredients in thirds and cherry syrup in halves to egg mixture. Stir in cherries. Pour into Pam–sprayed loaf pan. Bake at 350° for 40 to 42 minutes or until golden.

GLAZE:
1 cup 10X sugar
½ tablespoon Ultra Promise
  70% Less Fat

1½ tablespoons cherry syrup

Mix together 10X sugar and Ultra Promise. Add enough syrup to make thick paste. Cover bread with glaze.

Glazed Fruit Bread

1 (6–ounce) package dried
  peaches, chopped
1 cup raisins
1½ cups hot water
2 Egg Beaters

2 cups sugar
3½ cups self–rising flour
1 teaspoon salt
2 teaspoons vanilla

Combine peaches and raisins. Cover with hot water and set aside until cool. In a large bowl, combine Egg Beaters and sugar; beat. Stir in fruit. Add flour, salt and vanilla, mixing well. Pour into Pam–sprayed loaf pan. Bake at 300° for 1 hour. After 15 minutes cover top with aluminum foil to prevent over browning.

GLAZE:
¼ cup apricot nectar

¼ cup sugar

Combine and stir until smooth. With knife, cut slits into bread. Pour glaze over all while bread is warm.

Cranberry Bread I

2 cups self–rising flour
½ teaspoon salt
1 cup sugar
2 tablespoons Ultra Promise
  70% Less Fat

2 tablespoons Fleischmann's
  Fat Free Squeezable Spread
½ cup orange juice
1 Egg Beater
1½ cups fresh cranberries,
  halved

Mix together dry ingredients. In separate bowl, mix together Promise, Fleischmann's, orange juice and Egg Beaters. Add to dry ingredients. Stir in cranberries. Pour into Pam–sprayed loaf pan. Bake at 350° for 37 minutes.

Cranberry Bread II

6 tablespoons Ultra Promise
  70% Less Fat
¼ cup hot water
2 Egg Beaters

4 cups self–rising flour
2 cups sugar
1 cup orange juice
1 pound cranberries, chopped

Mix together Promise and hot water. In a separate bowl, mix together all dry ingredients; set aside. In a large bowl, add Egg Beaters, orange juice, water and Promise together; mix well. Add dry ingredients slowly. Fold in cranberries. Pour into 2 Pam–sprayed loaf pans. Bake at 350° for 40 minutes or until golden brown.

Glazed Orange–Poppy Seed Bread

3 cups self–rising flour
1½ cups skim milk
2¼ cups sugar
1½ teaspoons vanilla extract
1½ teaspoons butter flavoring
1½ teaspoons salt
3 Egg Beaters

8 tablespoons Ultra Promise
   70% Less Fat
2 tablespoons Fleischmann's
   Fat Free Squeezable Spread
1½ teaspoons poppy seeds
1½ teaspoons almond extract

Mix all ingredients together. Beat on medium speed for 2 minutes. Pour into 2 Pam–sprayed loaf pans. Bake at 350° for 45 minutes or until toothpick comes out clean.

GLAZE:
½ teaspoon butter extract
½ teaspoon vanilla extract
½ teaspoon almond extract

¾ cup sugar
¼ cup orange juice

Mix glaze until smooth. Pour over bread straight out of oven.

Lemon–Poppy Seed Bread

½ cup skim milk
2 lemons, fresh squeezed,
   divided
2½ teaspoons fresh lemon peel,
   divided
2 Egg Beaters

1 cup sugar
½ cup Weight Watcher's Fat
   Free Whipped Dressing
1½ cups self–rising flour
1 tablespoon poppy seeds
½ cup powdered sugar

Combine milk, 3 tablespoons lemon juice and 2 teaspoons peel; set aside. Beat Egg Beaters and sugar; stir in whipped dressing. Add flour and milk mixture alternately to whipped dressing mixture, beginning and ending with flour. Add poppy seeds. Pour batter into Pam–sprayed loaf pan. Bake at 350° for 35 minutes. Combine remaining lemon juice and rind with powdered sugar. Pour over warm bread. Cool for 10 minutes before removing from pan.

Glazed Pineapple Bread

2½ cups self–rising flour
1 cup sugar
2 Egg Beaters
1 small can crushed pineapple,
   undrained

2 tablespoons Ultra Promise
   70% Less Fat
3 tablespoons Fleischmann's
   Fat Free Squeezable Spread
2 tablespoons Karo syrup
1 tablespoon grated lemon peel

GLAZE:
½ cup pineapple juice
⅛ teaspoon coconut extract

¾ cup sugar

Combine dry ingredients. In separate bowl, combine Egg Beaters, pineapple with syrup, Promise, Fleischmann's, Karo and lemon peel. Stir into dry ingredients, blending only until all flour is moist. Pour into Pam–sprayed loaf pan. Bake at 350° for 30 minutes.

While bread is baking, combine all ingredients for glaze, stirring until sugar is dissolved. While bread is warm, cut holes with a sharp knife and pour glaze on top.

Orange Bread

2¼ cups self–rising flour
¾ cup sugar
3 tablespoons Ultra Promise
   70% Less Fat

1 Egg Beater
¾ cup orange juice
1 tablespoon grated fresh
   orange peel

Mix dry ingredients. Add remaining ingredients. Stir until mixture is moist, but not smooth. Pour into a Pam–sprayed loaf pan. Bake at 350° for 38 minutes. Top with aluminum foil after first 20 minutes to prevent over browning.

GLAZE (OPTIONAL):
2 to 3 tablespoons orange juice

1 cup powdered sugar

Blend orange juice into powdered sugar to make a thin glaze. While bread is warm, cut holes in cake with knife. Pour glaze over immediately.

Pineapple Bread

1 (8–ounce) can crushed
  pineapple, drained and ½ cup
  liquid reserved
2½ cups self–rising flour
⅓ cup brown sugar
¼ teaspoon ground cinnamon

3 tablespoons Ultra Promise
  70% Less Fat
5 tablespoons Fleischmann's
  Fat Free Squeezable Spread
½ cup sugar
1 Egg Beater
½ cup skim milk

Combine ½ cup flour, brown sugar, cinnamon, Promise and Fleischmann's; stir well. Combine rest of flour and sugar. In a separate bowl, combine Egg Beater, milk, pineapple and juice. Add liquid ingredients to dry ingredients. Stir just until moistened. Pour into a Pam–sprayed loaf pan. Bake at 350° for 35 minutes. After 20 minutes, cover with aluminum foil to prevent over browning.

Sweet Potato Bread

3 tablespoons Ultra Promise
  70% Less Fat
3 tablespoons Fleischmann's
  Fat Free Squeezable Spread
1 cup sugar, more or less
  depending on sweetness of
  potatoes
2 Egg Beaters
½ cup molasses

1 cup sweet potatoes, peeled,
  cooked and mashed
2 cups self–rising flour
½ teaspoon salt
½ teaspoon cinnamon
½ teaspoon nutmeg
½ teaspoon allspice
¼ teaspoon ground cloves
¼ cup raisins

Combine first 4 ingredients, beating until fluffy. Stir in molasses and potatoes. Combine dry ingredients and add to potato mixture. Add raisins. Blend well. Pour into Pam–sprayed loaf pan. Bake at 350° for 50 minutes. If over browning occurs, cover top with aluminum foil.

Pumpkin Bread

3 cups sugar
4 Egg Beaters
5 tablespoons Ultra Promise
   70% Less Fat
¾ cup Butter Buds Liquid
   (see page 50)
2 cups pumpkin

1 tablespoon soda
1½ teaspoons salt
1 teaspoon cinnamon
1 teaspoon nutmeg
3½ cups all–purpose flour
¾ cup water

Mix all ingredients in order given in mixing bowl, beating until well blended. Pour into 2 Pam–sprayed loaf pans. Bake at 350° for 55 minutes or until done.

Spiced Pumpkin Bread with Glaze

1 cup raisins
1 cup water
2 Egg Beaters
1 cup canned pumpkin pie
   filling
¼ cup water
¼ cup Butter Buds Liquid
   (see page 50)

1½ cups sugar
½ teaspoon salt
½ teaspoon nutmeg
½ teaspoon cinnamon
3 tablespoons Ultra Promise
   70% Less Fat

Combine raisins and water in small saucepan; bring to a boil; remove from heat and cool. Drain raisins. Mix Egg Beaters, pumpkin, water, Butter Buds Liquid, and Ultra Promise. Mix together dry ingredients. Stir pumpkin mixture into dry mixture. Add raisins; mix well. Pour into Pam–sprayed loaf pan. Bake at 350° for 50 minutes or until done.

GLAZE:
1 cup 10X sugar
1 tablespoon Ultra Promise
   70% Less Fat

¾ teaspoon cinnamon
1½ tablespoons skim milk

Mix together and top warm bread.

Banana Muffins

¼ cup Ultra Promise 70% Less
  Fat
¼ cup Butter Buds Liquid
  (see page 50)
1 cup sugar
1 Egg Beater

2 bananas, creamed
1 teaspoon soda
1 tablespoon water
1¾ cups self–rising flour
1 teaspoon vanilla

Mix Promise, Butter Buds Liquid and sugar. Add Egg Beater, then bananas. Dissolve soda in water and add to mixture. Gradually add flour, stirring well after each addition. Add vanilla. Spoon into Pam sprayed muffin tin. Bake at 375° for 16 minutes. Makes 12.

Bran Muffins

1 cup whole wheat flour
2 cups All–Bran cereal
1 teaspoon baking soda
½ teaspoon salt
½ cup molasses

1 Egg Beater
2 cups skim milk
1 cup raisins
2 tablespoons sugar

Mix cereal and milk and let stand. Meanwhile, mix together remaining ingredients. Add cereal and milk. Stir to moisten. Spoon into Pam–sprayed muffin tins. Bake at 375° for 20 minutes. Makes 18.

Blueberry–Orange Muffins

3 cups self–rising flour
1 cup sugar
½ teaspoon salt
2 cups blueberries
2 Egg Beaters

¾ cup skim milk
½ cup Ultra Promise, melted
1 tablespoon grated orange
  peel
½ cup orange juice

Mix together dry ingredients. Add blueberries and toss. In separate bowl add remaining ingredients. Pour liquid mixture into dry ingredients and stir. Fill Pam–sprayed muffin tins ⅔ full. Bake at 425° for 15 minutes. Makes 24 muffins.

Carrot Cake Muffins

1¾ cups self–rising flour
⅔ cup brown sugar
½ cup sugar
1 teaspoon cinnamon
⅛ teaspoon salt
¼ teaspoon allspice
¾ cup crushed pineapple in
   juice

3 tablespoons Ultra Promise
   70% Less Fat
¼ cup Fleischmann's Fat Free
   Squeezable Spread
1 Egg Beater
1½ teaspoons vanilla extract
2 cups carrots, shredded
½ cup raisins

Sift together dry ingredients; set aside. In small mixing bowl, mix together pineapple, Promise, Fleischmann's, Egg Beater, vanilla, carrots and raisins. Gently stir pineapple mixture into flour mixture until just moistened. Fill Pam–sprayed muffin tin ⅔ full. Bake at 400° for 11 minutes or until done.

Oatmeal Whole Wheat Muffins

1 cup oatmeal
½ teaspoon baking soda
1 cup non–fat buttermilk
1 Egg Beater
½ cup firmly packed brown
   sugar
¼ cup Ultra Promise 70% Less
   Fat
1 tablespoon Fleischmann's Fat
   Free Squeezable Spread

½ teaspoon salt
¼ teaspoon allspice
2 tablespoons sugar
1 tablespoon skim milk
½ teaspoon cinnamon
1 cup whole wheat flour
1 teaspoon baking powder
½ teaspoon vanilla extract

Soak oatmeal in buttermilk and baking soda for 5 minutes. Add Egg Beater and mix. Add sugars, Ultra Promise, Fleischmann's and milk; stir. Add remaining ingredients and stir only until moistened. Fill Pam–sprayed muffin tins ⅔ full. Bake at 400° for 18 to 20 minutes.

Orange Muffins with Sauce

½ cup Ultra Promise 70% Less
  Fat
1 cup sugar
2 Egg Beaters

⅔ cup non–fat buttermilk
2 cups self–rising flour
½ teaspoon salt
Orange Sauce II (See page 78)

Cream Promise and sugar. Add Egg Beaters. Mix well. Add dry ingredients and milk, alternately. Mix well. Bake at 375° for 16 minutes. While muffins are warm, spoon sauce over muffins while still in muffin tin. When cooled, remove from pan.

Pineapple–Banana Muffins

1 cup quick–cooking oats
1¼ cups self–rising flour
½ teaspoon cinnamon
2 Egg Beaters
½ cup brown sugar
1 teaspoon vanilla extract

¼ cup non–fat buttermilk
¼ cup Ultra Promise 70% Less
  Fat
1 (8–ounce) can crushed
  pineapple, undrained
1 cup diced banana

Combine first 3 ingredients in a bowl. In a separate bowl, mix Egg Beaters, sugar, vanilla, buttermilk and Ultra Promise. Pour all at once into dry mixture; stir only until moistened. Add pineapple and banana. Pour into Pam–sprayed muffin tin. Bake at 375° for 16 minutes.

Strawberry Muffins

1 Egg Beater
¼ cup Ultra Promise
¼ cup skim milk
¾ cup sugar

1 cup self–rising flour
½ cup sliced and sweetened
  frozen strawberries, thawed
Scant salt

Mix Egg Beater, Promise and milk together. In separate bowl, blend sugar, flour and salt; add to liquid mixture. Stir lightly. Add strawberries. Pour into Pam–sprayed muffin tin. Bake at 375° for 16 minutes. Makes 1 dozen.

Vanilla Muffins

2 cups sugar
4 Egg Beaters
4 cups self–rising flour
2 cups skim milk

1 tablespoon baking powder
½ cup Ultra Promise 70% Less Fat
1 tablespoon vanilla extract

Beat sugar and Egg Beaters together. Add flour, milk, baking powder, Promise and vanilla. Mix thoroughly. Bake at 350° for 9 to 10 minutes. Makes 36 muffins.

Buttermilk Corn Cakes

1 cup self–rising cornmeal
2 tablespoons sugar, optional

1 Egg Beater
1½ cups non–fat buttermilk

Combine dry ingredients. Add buttermilk, then Egg Beater. Cook in a 9–inch Pam–sprayed non–stick skillet. Cover until top of corn cakes appears "dry". Turn once, spraying pan with Pam. Makes 4 (9–inch) cakes.

Cornbread

1 cup self–rising cornmeal
⅛ cup self–rising flour
¼ teaspoon soda
2 tablespoons sugar or to taste
1 Egg Beater
½ cup non–fat buttermilk

½ cup skim milk
2 tablespoons Ultra Promise 70% Less Fat
2 tablespoons Fleischmann's Fat Free Squeezable Spread

Add together dry ingredients. Add Egg Beater, buttermilk and milk. Stir well. Add Promise and Fleischmann's. Pour into a Pam–sprayed iron skillet. Bake at 425° for 33 minutes.

Cornbread Squares

¾ cup self–rising cornmeal
1 cup self–rising flour
¼ cup sugar
1 cup fat–free sour cream
¼ cup skim milk

1 Egg Beater
2 tablespoons Ultra Promise
   70% Less Fat
1 teaspoon rosemary

Mix ingredients thoroughly. Pour into a Pam–sprayed 8 x 8–inch square baking dish. Bake at 425° for 20 minutes or until done.

Southern Cornbread

2 Egg Beaters
1 (8–ounce) can white cream
   style corn
1 cup fat–free sour cream

2 tablespoons Ultra Promise
   70% Less Fat
4 tablespoons Fleischmann's
   Fat Free Squeezable Spread
1 cup self–rising cornmeal

Combine Egg Beater, corn, sour cream, Promise, Fleischmann's, and cornmeal in bowl. Mix well. In a preheated, then Pam–sprayed iron skillet, pour batter. Bake at 400° for 20 minutes.

Caraway Rolls

1 package yeast
¼ cup warm water
1 tablespoon caraway seeds
1 cup fat–free cottage cheese

2 tablespoons sugar
1 teaspoon salt
1 Egg Beater
2⅓ cups self–rising flour

Dissolve yeast in water; add caraway seeds. Heat cottage cheese until lukewarm. Mix cottage cheese, sugar, salt and Egg Beater into yeast mixture. Slowly add flour, mixing until dough cleans bowl. Cover and let rise 1 hour. Stir down. Divide among 12 Pam–sprayed muffin tins. Cover and let rest 45 minutes. Bake at 350° for 15 minutes or until golden.

Butterhorns

1 cup skim milk
8 tablespoons Ultra Promise
   70% Less Fat
1 package yeast

3 Egg Beaters
½ cup sugar
½ teaspoon butter salt
4½ cups self–rising flour

Scald milk. Add Promise and cool to lukewarm. Dissolve yeast in milk and stir until dissolved. In a separate bowl add Egg Beaters, sugar and salt; beat. Add this mixture to yeast mixture. Add flour gradually. Knead, adding small amounts of flour, if needed, until you can handle it. Place in a Pam–sprayed bowl, cover, and let rise for 3 hours. Pat down and let rise until doubled. May be put in refrigerator until ready to use. When ready to use, divide into thirds and roll as for pie crust (about ⅛–inch thick). Cut into 16 pie–shaped wedges. Start at wide edge of each piece and roll. Bake at 350° for 10 minutes. Makes 48 rolls. Spray with I Can't Believe It's Not Butter spray after removing from oven.

Dinner Rolls

2 cups skim milk
½ cup Ultra Promise 70% Less
   Fat
½ cup sugar
6 cups self–rising flour

¾ teaspoon salt
1 package dry yeast
¼ cup water
1 egg white
1 tablespoon water

Combine milk, Promise and sugar. Heat until blended but do not boil. Cool until lukewarm. Mix together dry ingredients. Add to milk mixture. Dissolve yeast in warm water. Add to dough. Let rise in warm place until doubled. Add enough extra flour to make soft dough. Refrigerate and use as needed. When ready to use, shape as desired and let rise in warm place. Brush top with egg white and water mixture. Bake at 450° for 9 minutes.

Miracle Rolls

1 package yeast
1 cup non–fat buttermilk,
    warmed
¼ teaspoon soda
3 tablespoons sugar

3 tablespoons Ultra Promise
    70% Less Fat
2½ cups flour
1 egg white
1 tablespoon water

Place yeast in large bowl. Add buttermilk, soda, sugar and Promise, stirring until yeast is dissolved. Add flour. Stir until dough is of proper consistency, adding more flour if needed. Knead lightly, roll out and cut with biscuit cutter. Brush tops with egg white and water mixture. Cover and place in warm place for 1 hour. Bake at 375° for about 9 minutes.

Sour Cream Rolls

1 cup fat–free sour cream
½ cup sugar
1 teaspoon salt
½ cup Ultra Promise 70% Less
    Fat
½ cup warm water

2 packages yeast
2 Egg Beaters
4 cups self–rising flour
1 egg white
1 tablespoon water

Slightly melt sour cream in double boiler. Add ½ cup sugar, salt and Promise. Stir until Promise is melted. Cool to room temperature. Put yeast in water. Add sour cream mixture, Egg Beaters and flour to yeast. Stir until blended. Cover and refrigerate overnight. Next day: Bring dough to room temperature. Divide into 3 parts. Roll each part ½ inch thick. Cut with biscuit cutter. Brush tops with egg white and water mixture. Allow to rise until doubled. Bake at 375° for 12 minutes.

Break Apart Bread

2 cans biscuits (1 fat gram or
  less per biscuit)
1 medium bell pepper, finely
  chopped
1 small onion, finely chopped

2 slices Oscar Mayer bacon
Fat–free Parmesan cheese
I Can't Believe It's Not Butter
  spray
Pam butter spray

Sauté peppers and onions in Pam–butter spray; set aside. Fry bacon until crisp; drain well by pressing bacon between paper towels to remove as much grease as possible. Crumble and set aside.

Quarter biscuits, 1 can at a time; spray with Pam butter spray and lightly sprinkle with Parmesan cheese. Place in a Pam–sprayed bundt pan. Sprinkle pepper, onion and bacon over biscuits. Add more Parmesan cheese. Place remaining can of biscuits on top of this. Generously top with Parmesan cheese. Bake at 350° for 30 minutes or until done.

Caramel Pull Aparts

1 can lowfat biscuits, cut into
  fourths
⅓ cup sugar

1 teaspoon cinnamon
¼ cup No–Cook Caramel Sauce
  (see page 77)

In a small mixing bowl mix together sugar and cinnamon. Roll the cut biscuits in sugar mixture. Place in a Pam–sprayed loaf pan. Pour ¼ cup of No–Cook Caramel Sauce over all. Bake at 325° for 20 minutes or until golden. Spoon additional sauce over top after removing from oven.

Cheesy Spoon Bread

2 cups skim milk
½ cup yellow self–rising
  cornmeal
1 tablespoon Ultra Promise
  70% Less Fat

Scant salt
2 Egg Beaters
½ cup fat–free Cheddar cheese,
  grated
2 egg whites, beaten

Warm milk in saucepan—DO NOT BOIL. Stir in cornmeal, Promise and salt and let cook until slightly thickened. Add Egg Beaters and cheese; beat to keep smooth. Add stiff beaten egg whites and fold into cornmeal mixture. Pour into a Pam–sprayed casserole dish. Bake at 375° for 40 minutes.

Herb Loaf

1 (1–pound) loaf frozen white
  Kroger bread dough

3 tablespoons spaghetti sauce
  mix, dry
Butter flavor Pam spray

While bread is frozen, spray with Pam spray and roll in spaghetti sauce mix, making sure all surface is covered. Follow instructions on wrapper and bake bread accordingly. Watch to make sure over browning does not occur. If so, cover with aluminum foil.

VARIATIONS: Substitute taco seasoning for spaghetti seasoning.

Herbed Rolls

Rhodes Fat Free Lite frozen
  dinner rolls
Garlic powder

Oregano
Fat–free Parmesan cheese

Roll frozen dough mixture in each of the ingredients above. Let thaw and cook according to directions.

Italian Herbed Rolls

Rhodes Bake N Serve Lite Fat
  Free Bread dough, frozen

1 package McCormick
  spaghetti sauce mix
Butter flavor Pam spray

Use microwave thaw directions. After removing from microwave, spray with Pam spray. Roll dough in spaghetti sauce seasoning mix until thoroughly covered. Let rise and bake according to package directions.

Orange Biscuit Ring

½ cup sugar
1½ tablespoons grated orange
  rind

2 (12–ounce) cans biscuits (1 fat
  gram or less per biscuit)
Pam butter spray

Combine sugar and orange rind. Spray biscuits, front and back, with Pam butter spray. Cut biscuits into fourths. Roll into sugar mixture. Drop biscuits in a Pam–sprayed tube pan. Bake at 350° for 30 minutes or until golden browned. Cool for 5 minutes and invert on serving plate.

GLAZE:
½ cup 10X sugar
1 tablespoon Fleischmann's Fat
  Free Squeezable Spread

2 teaspoons orange juice

Mix 10X sugar with Fleischmann's. Add orange juice and mix well. Pour onto biscuits while still warm.

Apple Pancakes

2 cups self–rising flour
2 cups skim milk
2 Egg Beaters
Pinch of salt
½ teaspoon vanilla extract

3 medium apples, peeled, cored
   and sliced
1 cup sugar
Allspice

Combine first 5 ingredients in mixing bowl; blend until smooth. Set aside.

For each pancake use ¼ cup batter. Heat non–stick 6–inch skillet over medium heat. Spray with Pam butter spray. Pour batter onto skillet. Cook until partially set but still a little liquid. Cover with apple slices. Flip pancake, sprayed with Pam spray. Sprinkle browned side with 1 teaspoon sugar. Spray sugared side with Pam butter spray and flip again. Repeat until both sides are golden brown and sugar glazed. After pancakes are done, sprinkle one side with 1 teaspoon sugar and lightly dust with allspice. Makes 10 (6–inch) pancakes.

Apple–Pineapple Pancakes

1 cup self–rising flour
2 Egg Beaters
½ cup skim milk
1 apple, peeled, cored and
   diced well

1 cup crushed pineapple, well
   drained
3 tablespoons sugar
¼ teaspoon vanilla extract
10X sugar

Combine all ingredients well; let set for 15 minutes.

Pour ¼ cup of batter into a hot Pam–sprayed non–stick skillet. Cook until golden. Before turning pancake over, spray pan with Pam again. Cook until golden. Sprinkle with 10X sugar.

Blueberry Pancakes

1 cup whole wheat flour
1 cup all–purpose flour
4 teaspoons baking powder
2 tablespoons sugar
¼ teaspoon cinnamon
2 cups skim milk
1 Egg Beater
2 tablespoons orange juice, fresh

3 tablespoons Ultra Promise 70% Less Fat
1 tablespoon Fleischmann's Fat Free Squeezable Spread
⅛ teaspoon vanilla extract
½ cup blueberries
Powdered sugar

Combine dry ingredients in large bowl; mix well. Stir in milk, Egg Beater, orange juice, Promise, Fleischmann's and vanilla; do not over mix. Fold in blueberries. Cook at 400° on Pam–sprayed griddle using ¼ cup per pancake. Cook until golden brown. Spray with Pam before turning. Cook until done. Sprinkle with powdered sugar and serve. Makes 20 pancakes.

Whole Wheat Pancakes

3 Egg Beaters
2 cups skim milk
¼ cup Ultra Promise 70% Less Fat
¼ cup honey
¼ cup sugar

2½ cups whole wheat flour
5 teaspoons baking powder
1 teaspoon cinnamon
1 teaspoon ground nutmeg
¼ teaspoon salt

In an 8–cup mixing bowl, combine first 5 ingredients. Blend together remaining ingredients. Add remaining ingredients to egg mixture. Cook on a Pam–sprayed griddle, using ¼ cup per pancake. Cook until golden brown, spray pancake with Pam and flip. Cook until golden brown and done.

Sour Cream Pancakes

1 cup self–rising flour
2 tablespoons sugar
1 Egg Beater
1 cup skim milk

¼ cup fat–free sour cream
2 tablespoons Fleischmann's
    Fat Free Squeezable Spread
¼ teaspoon butter salt

Add all ingredients; mix well. Fry on hot Pam–sprayed griddle until golden brown. Serve with warm syrup.

Yeast Pancakes

2½ cups self–rising flour
½ cup sugar
1½ teaspoons yeast
1¾ cups warm water

½ teaspoon soda
½ teaspoon salt
¾ cup skim milk

Blend flour, sugar, yeast and warm water together; cover with Pam–sprayed plastic. Set aside for 1 hour. Add soda and salt to warm milk and stir into batter. (Batter needs to be runny, so a little more milk may be added.) Cover again for 30 minutes. Heat Pam–sprayed griddle and pour ¼ cup batter to make each pancake. Gently cook for about 10 minutes or until set and bubbles have burst. Serve warm with syrup or honey.

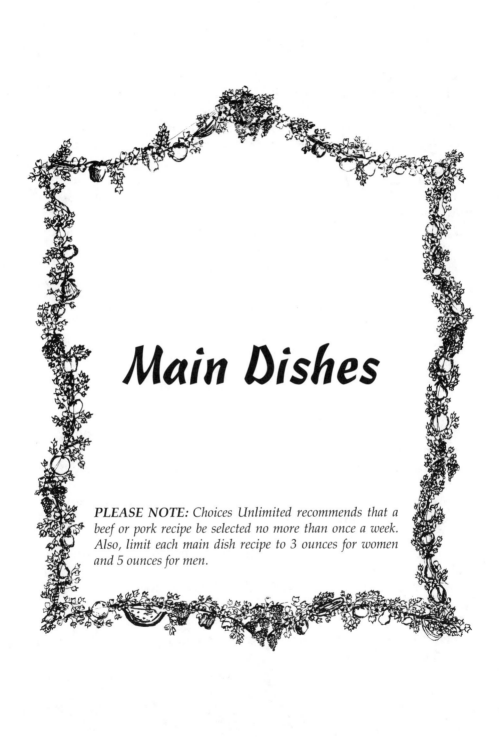

Main Dishes

PLEASE NOTE: *Choices Unlimited recommends that a beef or pork recipe be selected no more than once a week. Also, limit each main dish recipe to 3 ounces for women and 5 ounces for men.*

Apricot Chicken

2 whole chicken breasts,
    skinned, boned and halved
Juice of 1 lemon
Allspice
½ cup onion, thinly sliced

1 teaspoon ground ginger
½ cup orange juice
¼ teaspoon black pepper
Salt to taste
1 cup dried apricots

Marinate chicken in lemon juice 30 minutes to an hour. Sprinkle chicken with allspice and cook in a Pam–sprayed non–stick skillet until done and browned. Sauté onion in Pam–sprayed skillet and add to chicken. Add remaining ingredients, stir. Cover; bring to a simmer for 15 to minutes. May be served with rice.

Baked Chicken Supreme

4 chicken breasts, split and
    boned
1 teaspoon salt
¼ teaspoon pepper
2 teaspoons cornstarch
¼ cup green onions, mixed
¼ cup chicken broth

¾ cup white wine
½ pound fresh mushrooms,
    sliced
1 tablespoon dried thyme or to
    taste
2 cups seedless white grapes

In a non–stick, Pam–sprayed skillet, brown chicken, sprinkling with salt and pepper. Arrange chicken close together in shallow pan. Sauté onions in a Pam–sprayed skillet. Stir in broth, wine, thyme and cornstarch. Pour over chicken. Cover and bake at 350° for 1 hour. Sauté mushrooms in a non–stick, Pam–sprayed skillet. Add to chicken along with grapes. Cover and cook an additional 10 minutes. May be served with rice.

Barbara's Chicken and Asparagus Casserole

6 chicken breasts, boneless and halved
1 carrot
1 celery rib
1 bay leaf
2 (#2) cans asparagus, drained
1 can Campbell's Healthy Request cream of mushroom soup
1 can Campbell's Healthy Request cream of chicken soup
¾ cup Weight Watcher's Fat Free Whipped Dressing
1 small jar pimentos, drained

Cook chicken breasts with carrot, celery and bay leaf until done. Discard vegetables and bay leaf; dice chicken. Layer in a Pam–sprayed casserole dish. Top with asparagus. Combine remaining ingredients; mix well. Cover asparagus. Bake at 325° for 35 minutes or until bubbly.

Butter Roasted Chicken

8 chicken breast halves, boned and skinned
¼ cup Butter Buds Liquid (see page 50)
¼ cup Fleischmann's Fat Free Squeezable Spread
Juice of 2 lemons
2 teaspoons salt
1 teaspoon pepper
3 teaspoons paprika
½ teaspoon brown sugar
Dash Tabasco
⅛ teaspoon powdered rosemary

In a small saucepan place all ingredients, omitting chicken. Stir well over low heat until seasonings are well blended. Brush sauce over chicken. Place in a shallow pan. Roast in 325° oven for 2 hours, basting with sauce every 15 minutes.

Cheesy Chicken Bake

1 cup celery, chopped
1 green pepper, chopped
1 cup onion, chopped
1 (7–ounce) can mushrooms,
    drained
2 cans Campbell's Healthy
    Request cream of mushroom
    soup

2 cups Fat Free Cheddar cheese,
    shredded
1 (16–ounce) package spaghetti
    noodles
2 chicken bouillon cubes
4 chicken breasts, boned,
    skinned, cooked and drained
Salt and pepper to taste

Sauté celery, pepper and onion in a non–stick, Pam–sprayed skillet. Add mushrooms, soup and cheese. Cook noodles according to package directions but add bouillon cubes; drain when done. In a Pam–sprayed casserole dish, make 2 layers by layering noodles, chicken and soup mixture; repeat. Bake uncovered at 350° for 25 minutes or until bubbly.

Chicken and Asparagus Casserole

6 chicken breasts, skinned and
    boned
2 carrots, quartered
2 celery ribs, quartered
1 to 2 bay leaves
Salt and pepper to taste
2 (#2) cans asparagus, drained
1 can Campbell's Healthy
    Request cream of mushroom
    soup

1 can Campbell's Healthy
    Request cream of chicken
    soup
¾ cup Weight Watcher's Fat
    Free Whipped Dressing
1 small jar pimentos
Paprika

Cook chicken breasts with carrots, celery, bay leaves, salt and pepper until done. Drain and dice chicken. Use cooked carrots and celery elsewhere. Discard bay leaves. Place asparagus in the bottom of a Pam–sprayed casserole dish; top with prepared chicken. Mix together the soups, whipped dressing and pimentos. Spoon mixture over chicken. Sprinkle top with paprika. Bake at 325° for 30 minutes or until bubbly.

Chicken and Dressing Casserole

3 chicken breasts, boned,
  skinned, cooked and diced
1 can Campbell's Healthy
  Request cream of celery soup
1 can Campbell's Healthy
  Request cream of chicken soup

1 small package Pepperidge
  Farm dressing mix
1¼ cups chicken broth
½ cup Butter Buds Liquid
  (see page 50)

Place cooked chicken in the bottom of a Pam–sprayed casserole dish. Combine soups. Spoon soups over chicken. Sprinkle dressing mix over soup. Mix broth and Butter Buds Liquid and pour over all. Bake at 350° for 35 minutes.

Fried Chicken and Gravy

CHICKEN:
1 cup corn flake crumbs
1 teaspoon paprika
½ teaspoon garlic powder
¾ teaspoon parsley flakes
¼ teaspoon ground thyme

¼ teaspoon ground red pepper
¼ cup nonfat buttermilk
6 chicken breasts, boneless,
  skinless

Combine first 6 ingredients in a bowl. Brush both sides of chicken breasts with buttermilk. Roll in corn flake mixture. Bake, uncovered, on a Pam–sprayed cookie sheet at 400° for 20 minutes or until completely done.

GRAVY:
1 can Campbell's Healthy
  Request cream of chicken
  soup

½ cup evaporated skimmed
  milk

Combine soup and milk. Arrange cooked chicken in a Pam–sprayed casserole dish. Pour soup mixture over all. Cook at 350° for 20 minutes or until bubbly. Serve hot.

VARIATIONS: Campbell's Healthy Request cream of mushroom soup or Campbell's cream of celery soup may be used in place of low–fat cream of chicken soup.

Chicken Breasts in Peach Sauce

2 whole chicken breasts, split,
  skinned and boned

SAUCE:
½ cup peach preserves
4 teaspoons Dijon mustard
1 tablespoon Ultra Promise
  70% Less Fat

1 tablespoon Fleischmann's Fat
  Free Squeezable Spread
1 teaspoon sugar

In a small saucepan, mix sauce ingredients and heat until blended. Arrange chicken breasts in a shallow Pam–sprayed casserole dish. Pour sauce over chicken. Cover and bake at 350° for 15 minutes. Uncover and bake an additional 15 minutes. Serve over pasta or rice.

Chicken Breasts Supreme

8 chicken breasts, skinless,
  boneless
½ pint fat–free sour cream

1 can Campbell's Healthy
  Request cream of mushroom
  soup
1 cup sherry
Paprika

Combine sour cream, soup and sherry. In a Pam–sprayed casserole dish, place chicken in a single layer. Pour soup mixture over chicken. Bake at 350° for 1 hour and 15 minutes, or until done. Sprinkle with paprika before serving.

Chicken Casserole

1½ cooked chickens, diced
1 can water chestnuts, diced
1 can asparagus, drained
1 green pepper, diced
1 (4–ounce) can mushrooms

1 can Campbell's Healthy
  Request cream of mushroom
  soup
¼ cup skimmed milk

Layer first 5 ingredients, in order given, in Pam–sprayed casserole dish. Mix milk and soup together. Pour over all. Bake at 350° fro 25 minutes or until bubbly.

Chicken Broccoli Casserole

2 (10–ounce) packages frozen
   broccoli
4 chicken breasts, boned,
   skinned and diced
1 cup Weight Watcher's Fat
   Free Whipped Dressing
2 cans Campbell's Healthy
   Request cream of mushroom
   soup

1 small jar pimentos
1 teaspoon fresh lemon juice
¼ to ½ teaspoon curry
½ cup fat–free Cheddar cheese
½ cup fat–free bread crumbs
½ tablespoon Ultra Promise
   70% Less Fat

Prepare broccoli according to package directions; drain. Place broccoli in the bottom of a Pam–sprayed casserole dish. Top with prepared chicken. In separate bowl, combine whipped dressing, soup, pimentos, lemon juice, curry and cheese. Pour over chicken. Melt Promise; pour over crumbs and toss well. Spread crumbs evenly on top. Bake at 350° for 25 to 30 minutes or until bubbly.

Chicken Divine

6 chicken breasts, skinned,
   boned and halved
¼ cup Fleischmann's Fat Free
   Squeezable Spread
1 (10¾–ounce) can Campbell's
   Healthy Request cream of
   chicken soup
2½ tablespoons onion, grated

1 teaspoon salt
Pepper to taste
½ tablespoon dried parsley
   flakes
½ teaspoon celery flakes
⅛ teaspoon thyme
1⅓ cups water
1 cup Minute rice

Cook chicken and cut into bite–sized pieces; set aside. Combine Fleischmann's, soup, seasoning and water in saucepan, and heat, stirring occasionally, to a boil. Spread uncooked rice in a 1½ quart Pam–sprayed casserole. Pour all but ½ cup of soup mixture over rice. Stir to moisten. Top with chicken. Then add remaining soup mixture. Bake covered at 375° for 30 minutes or until chicken is tender.

Chicken Dijon

6 chicken breasts, boned and
  skinned
1 (16–ounce) jar Dijon mustard
1 (16–ounce) carton fat–free
  sour cream

Seasoned bread crumbs
Fleischmann's Fat Free
  Squeezable Spread

Rinse chicken and pat dry. Spread both sides liberally with Fleischmann's, mustard and sour cream. Roll (or sprinkle) heavily with crumbs. Cover with foil. Bake at 400° for 30 minutes. Remove top and bake at 450° for 15 minutes.

Chicken Fajitas

MARINADE:
¼ cup water
⅓ cup red wine vinegar
1 teaspoon brown sugar
1 teaspoon dried oregano
¼ teaspoon garlic powder

¼ teaspoon minced onion
¼ teaspoon lemon pepper
½ teaspoon salt
juice of 1 lime

FILLING:
4 chicken breasts, boneless and
  skinless
1 large onion

1 each red, yellow and green
  peppers

TOPPINGS:
10 (8–inch) flour tortillas
Salsa
Fat–free sour cream

1 cup fat–free Cheddar cheese,
  grated

Cut chicken into strips. Mix together marinade. Add chicken strips and refrigerate 4 to 8 hours. After marinating, broil chicken strips 4 to 6 minutes on each side, brushing with marinade after turning. In a non–stick, Pam–sprayed skillet, sauté peppers and onions until crisp–tender. Fill tortillas with chicken, filling and toppings.

Chicken Lasagna

12 lasagna noodles, cooked and
  drained
1 can Campbell's Healthy
  Request cream of mushroom
  soup
⅔ cup skim milk
1 (8–ounce) package fat–free
  mozzarella cheese, shredded
1 carton fat–free cottage cheese

½ cup onions, finely chopped
½ cup green peppers, finely
  chopped
1 teaspoon dried parsley
2 cups chicken, cooked and
  diced
1 cup bread crumbs
I Can't Believe It's Not Butter
  Spray

Mix together soup, milk, mozzarella cheese and cottage cheese. Heat until cheese melts; set aside. Mix together onions, peppers and parsley; set aside. In a 9 x 13–inch Pam–sprayed casserole dish, layer noodles, cheese mixture, onion, pepper, and chicken. Repeat until dish is full. Cover with bread crumbs and spray with butter spray. Bake at 325° for 30 minutes or until bubbly. Let stand 5 minutes.

Waikiki Chicken

6 chicken breasts, skinned,
  boned and halved
Fat–free French dressing
1 (20–ounce) can pineapple
  chunks
½ cup chicken broth
2 tablespoons soy sauce
3 tablespoons lemon juice

1 tablespoon cornstarch
1 (10–ounce) package frozen
  pea pods, cooked
1 (5–ounce) can water
  chestnuts, drained and sliced
⅓ cup green onions, chopped
Salt and pepper to taste

Brush chicken with dressing. Place in Pam–sprayed baking pan. Bake at 450° for 10 minutes. Drain pineapple, reserve juice. Mix pineapple juice, broth and soy sauce. Add lemon juice to cornstarch and stir into pineapple juice mixture. Pour over chicken breasts. Reduce heat to 350° and bake about 45 minutes or until chicken is lightly browned and tender. Combine pineapple chunks, cooked peas, water chestnuts, onion, salt and pepper. Sprinkle over chicken, heat, then serve.

Chicken Tetrazzini

2 boneless, skinless chicken
  breasts
2 teaspoons pepper
1 (9–ounce) package angel hair
  pasta
2 tablespoons Ultra Promise
  70% Fat Free
2 tablespoons Fleischmann's
  Fat Free Squeezable Spread

¾ pound mushrooms, sliced
¼ cup flour
½ teaspoon salt
1 cup evaporated skimmed
  milk
¼ cup sherry
½ cup fat–free Parmesan cheese
3 cups chicken broth

Place chicken and pepper in water and simmer, covered, until done. Cook angel hair in 3 cups chicken broth for 45 minutes. Remove angel hair, reserving 2 cups of broth. Place angel hair in a Pam–sprayed 2–quart shallow baking dish. Cut chicken into bite–size pieces. In a non–stick, Pam–sprayed skillet, sauté mushrooms. Stir flour into Ultra Promise and Fleischmann's. Add broth and stir until smooth. Add evaporated skimmed milk and sherry. Heat slowly, stirring until thickened. Remove from heat; add chicken. Pour over angel hair and sprinkle with cheese. Bake at 350° for 20 minutes or until bubbly.

Company Chicken

4 chicken breasts, skinned,
  boned and split
¼ cup Fleischmann's Fat Free
  Squeezable Spread
Salt to taste
Pepper to taste
1 cup dry white wine

1 cup chicken broth
2 ounces port wine
1 cup evaporated skimmed
  milk
½ teaspoon rosemary
1 tablespoon cornstarch
1 tablespoon water

Brown chicken in a Pam–sprayed, non–stick skillet; add salt and pepper. Add white wine, broth and Fleischmann's. Simmer for 45 minutes or until done. Remove chicken. Add port wine, milk and seasonings; stir until smooth. Mix cornstarch and water; add to broth mixture, stirring until thickened. Pour over chicken. Serve with rice.

Cissy's Enchiladas

1 pound Butterball's Fat Free
  turkey breast, cooked
1 package Lawry's burrito
  seasoning mix
¾ cup hot water
Mission Fat Free flour tortillas

Fat–free sour cream
Onions, diced
Fat–free Cheddar cheese,
  shredded
1 (10–ounce) can green chili
  enchilada sauce

Cook ground turkey, add seasoning packet and water. Cook until liquid is gone. Fill flour tortillas by spooning sour cream in middle of tortilla. Layer with meat mixture, onions, cheese and enchilada sauce. Roll tortilla and place in a Pam–sprayed dish that has a very thin layer of enchilada sauce on the bottom. Repeat until all is used up. Bake, covered at 350° or until thoroughly hot. Before serving, pour a small amount of enchilada sauce over the top of each one.

Chicken With Pineapple

2 whole chicken breasts,
  skinned, boned and halved
1½ cups pineapple juice
1 tablespoon brown sugar
2 tablespoons soy sauce
2 tablespoons honey
1 fresh pineapple cut into
  bite–size pieces

1 green pepper, cut into strips
1 red pepper, cut into strips
½ cup water chestnuts, sliced
1 tablespoon Fleischmann's Fat
  Free Squeezable Spread
Rice

Make a marinade out of pineapple juice, brown sugar, soy sauce and honey. Place chicken in a nonmetallic dish and cover with marinade. Refrigerate several hours or overnight. Sauté peppers in a Pam–sprayed, non–stick skillet until tender crisp; remove and set aside. Cook chicken 2 to 3 minutes per side. Pour marinade over chicken and simmer 15 minutes. Add pineapple, peppers, water chestnuts and Ultra Promise. Cook an additional 5 minutes. Serve over rice.

Company Crab and Chicken Spectacular

1 (7½–ounce) can crabmeat
3 chicken breasts, boned,
  skinned, cooked and sliced
½ cup mushrooms, sliced
¼ cup onion, chopped
3 tablespoons Fleischmann's
  Fat Free Squeezable Spread
3 tablespoons flour
½ teaspoon salt
⅛ teaspoon white pepper
1½ cups chicken broth
½ cup dry white wine
2 Egg Beaters
1 cup peas, cooked
⅓ cup evaporated skimmed
  milk
¼ cup fat–free Parmesan cheese

Drain and flake crab; set aside. Place chicken in a Pam–sprayed baking pan; set aside. Sauté mushrooms and onions in a non–stick, Pam–sprayed skillet; set aside. In same non–stick skillet, blend in flour, salt and pepper. Gradually add broth and wine, whisking continually. Cook until thickened. Gradually add Egg Beaters and blend thoroughly. Cook an additional 2 minutes. Remove from heat. Stir in mushrooms, onion, peas and crab. Fold in evaporated milk. Pour sauce over chicken in casserole. Sprinkle with Parmesan cheese. Bake at 325° for 20 minutes or until bubbly.

Creamed Chicken Over Toast Points

1 tablespoon Butter Buds
  powder
2 tablespoons cornstarch
1½ cups evaporated skimmed
  milk
3 cups chicken breasts, cooked
  and cubed
1 can Campbell's Healthy
  Request cream of mushroom
  soup
1 tablespoon pimento
3 teaspoons dry basil or to taste
Salt to taste
Fat–free Cheddar cheese,
  shredded
Green onion, diced

Mix first 3 ingredients and cook over medium heat, stirring constantly until thickened. Stir in chicken, soup, basil and pimento, cooking until thoroughly hot. Serve over toast points. Sprinkle with cheese and onion.

Creole Chicken

2 whole chicken breasts, skinned, boned and halved
Ground cloves
⅔ cup onion, chopped
½ cup celery, diced
½ cup green pepper, diced
½ teaspoon garlic, minced
½ teaspoon pepper
¼ teaspoon ground red pepper
½ teaspoon salt
1 teaspoon thyme
1 bay leaf
1 (16–ounce) can stewed tomatoes
1 teaspoon sugar
Rice

Lightly sprinkle chicken with cloves. Brown chicken in a Pam–sprayed, non–stick skillet. Remove; set aside. Clean skillet and spray with Pam spray. Sauté onion, celery and green pepper. Add tomatoes and seasonings. Cook 5 minutes. Add chicken, cover and slowly simmer 15 minutes. Remove bay leaf. Serve over rice.

Crock Pot Chicken Tetrazzini

4 boneless, skinless chicken breast halves cut into 2–inch strips
1 chicken bouillon cube
1 cup water
½ cup dry white wine
1 cup onion, diced
½ teaspoon salt
¼ teaspoon dried thyme
¼ teaspoon pepper
1 tablespoon dried parsley
1 small can mushrooms
3 tablespoons cornstarch
¼ cup water
½ cup evaporated skimmed milk
8 ounces spaghetti, broken into thirds, cooked and drained
⅓ cup Parmesan cheese

In a crock pot, combine chicken, bouillon cube, water, wine, onion, salt, thyme, pepper and parsley. Cover and cook on low for 4 hours. Turn to high and add mushrooms. In a small bowl add cornstarch and water; stir into crock pot and cook for 20 minutes. Stir in evaporated skimmed milk and cooked spaghetti. Cook an additional 5 to 10 minutes. Top with Parmesan cheese.

Easy Mustard–Honey Chicken

¼ cup Fleischmann's Fat Free
  Squeezable Spread
½ cup honey
¼ cup prepared mustard

1 teaspoon curry
½ teaspoon salt
4 large chicken breast halves,
  skinned

Mix first 5 ingredients together. Place chicken in Pam–sprayed baking dish and bake at 375° for 20 minutes, basting once. Turn chicken and bake 20 to 30 minutes until fork tender, basting twice.

Farm–style Supper

1 box low–fat macaroni and
  cheese
¼ cup Fleischmann's Fat Free
  Squeezable Spread
¼ cup skim milk

8 ounces fat–free turkey
  sausage, sliced
1 (8–ounce) can lima beans
  with juice

Cook macaroni noodles in salted water. Drain. Add Fleischmann's, skim milk and cheese sauce mix; mix well. Add remaining ingredients. Bake at 350° for 30 minutes or until thoroughly heated.

Herb Batter "Fried" Chicken

2 tablespoons fat–free Italian
  dressing
½ cup fat–free ranch dressing
1 Egg Beater

6 chicken breasts, skinned
½ cup flour
2 cups corn flake crumbs

Combine dressings and Egg Beater; set aside. Rinse chicken and pat dry. Roll chicken in flour, dip into dressing mixture. Roll in corn flake crumbs. Place on a foil–lined baking pan. Bake at 350° for 20 to 30 minutes.

Golden Chicken with Grapes

2 chicken breasts, boned,
skinned and halved
1 can Campbell's Healthy
Request cream of mushroom
soup
2 medium sweet potatoes,
peeled and cut into ½–inch
slices

¼ cup water
½ teaspoon salt
⅛ teaspoon grated nutmeg
Salt and pepper to taste
1 cup red seedless grapes,
halved

In a non–stick, Pam–sprayed skillet, brown chicken. Remove chicken and combine remaining ingredients omitting grapes. Add chicken. Cover and cook at low heat for 45 minutes or until done. Stir occasionally. Or may be baked at 350° for 45 minutes. Add grapes during last 10 minutes.

Hot Chicken Salad Casserole

1½ cups rice
⅔ cup Weight Watcher's Fat
Free Whipped Dressing
1 can Campbell's Healthy
Request cream of chicken
soup
½ can Campbell's Healthy
Request cream of mushroom
soup
1 small can mushrooms,
drained

2½ cups chicken, cooked and
diced
3 tablespoons onion, grated
1 cup celery, diced
¼ cup green peppers
3 tablespoons pimentos
3 hard–boiled egg whites
2 tablespoons lemon juice
1 tablespoon soy sauce
Baked Lay's potato chips,
crushed

Cook rice according to package directions. Combine all ingredients together except for potato chips. Pour into a Pam–sprayed casserole dish. Top with a sparse layer of crushed potato chips. Bake at 350° for 30 minutes.

Jane Proctor's Chicken and Ham

6 chicken breast halves, boned
  and skinned
6 thin ham slices
6 fat–free American cheese slices
2 Egg Beaters

2 cups bread crumbs
  (see page 161)
1 can Campbell's Healthy
  Request cream of celery soup,
  undiluted

Pound chicken breasts flat. Place a slice of ham and cheese on each breast; roll; secure with a toothpick. Dip into Egg Beater and roll in bread crumbs. Slightly brown in a non–stick, Pam–sprayed skillet. Place in a Pam–sprayed casserole dish. Cover with soup. Bake at 350° for 1 hour.

Katie's Poppy Seed Chicken

8 chicken breasts, cooked and
  chopped
2 cans Campbell's Healthy
  Request cream of chicken
  soup
1½ pints fat–free sour cream

2 tablespoons poppy seeds
16 reduced fat Ritz crackers
16 fat–free crackers
I Can't Believe It's Not Butter
  spray

Mix soup and sour cream; add poppy seeds and set aside. Crumble crackers; set aside. Layer in a 9 x 13–inch Pam–sprayed casserole dish with half of the sauce on bottom, half of the chicken in middle, and half of the bread crumbs on top. Spray generously with butter spray. Repeat. Bake at 350° for 30 minutes.

Linda's Chicken Savannah

6 chicken breasts, boned,
  skinned and halved
¼ cup Butter Buds Liquid
  (see page 50)

¼ cup Fleischmann's Fat Free
  Squeezable Spread
1 package onion soup mix
6 ounces barbecue sauce

Mix together Butter Buds Liquid, Fleischmann's, soup mix and sauce, mixing thoroughly. Coat chicken with sauce. Bake, covered, at 350° for 1 hour. Baste chicken with remaining sauce.

Mexican Chicken

2 whole chicken breasts,
skinned, boned and halved

Spanish Rice (see page 273)

MARINADE:
1 cup picante sauce
¼ cup fresh lime juice
1 tablespoon Dijon mustard

½ teaspoon sugar
2 teaspoons fresh cilantro,
chopped

Marinate chicken in a shallow, nonmetallic dish for at least 1 hour, turning once. Cook chicken in a Pam–sprayed, non–stick skillet until done. Pour marinade over chicken. Cover and slowly simmer 15 minutes. Serve over Spanish Rice.

Mrs. Higg's Chicken and Broccoli Casserole

3 chicken breasts, cooked and
diced
2 (10–ounce) packages broccoli,
cooked and drained
1 cup Weight Watcher's Fat
Free Whipped Dressing
2 cans Campbell's Healthy
Request cream of mushroom
soup

1 small jar pimentos, drained
2 teaspoons lemon juice
½ teaspoon curry
½ cup fat–free Cheddar cheese,
shredded
½ cup soft bread crumbs
1 tablespoon Ultra Promise
70% Less Fat, melted

Layer broccoli in a Pam–sprayed 9 x 13–inch casserole dish; cover with chicken. In a separate bowl mix together whipped dressing, soup, pimentos, lemon juice, curry and cheese. Cover chicken with soup mixture. Top with bread crumbs and melted Promise. Bake at 350° for 30 minutes or until bubbly.

Orange Chicken

6 chicken breast halves,
skinned and boned
½ cup green onions, sliced
1 (6–ounce) can orange juice
concentrate, thawed

1 teaspoon tarragon
Pinch of salt
2 tablespoons cornstarch
2 tablespoons water

Sauté onions in a non–stick, Pam–sprayed skillet. Place chicken in large skillet. Combine onions, orange juice, tarragon and salt; pour over chicken. Cover and simmer 30 minutes. Remove chicken. Combine cornstarch and water. Add to skillet and cook until thick. Pour over chicken. Serve hot.

Orange Spicy Chicken

⅓ cup orange marmalade
⅓ cup hot barbecue sauce
2 tablespoons Worcestershire
sauce

2 tablespoons lemon juice
4 chicken breasts, skinned,
deboned and halved
Salt and pepper to taste

Mix together first 4 ingredients. Place chicken in a Pam–sprayed baking dish. Lightly sprinkle with salt and pepper. Pour sauce over chicken. Cover. Bake in 350° oven for 30 minutes. Uncover. Continue baking for 45 to 60 minutes or until golden brown.

Thyme Chicken

4 chicken breast, deboned,
skinless and split
½ teaspoon garlic powder
1 small green pepper, sliced
1 (1–pound) can tomatoes

1 medium onion, thinly sliced
½ cup white wine
¾ teaspoon salt
¼ teaspoon thyme
⅛ teaspoon marjoram

Place chicken in a Pam–sprayed, non–stick skillet and cook until done. Sauté onions and peppers in a Pam–sprayed, non–stick skillet. Add to chicken. Add remaining ingredients. Cover and simmer for 25 minutes or until tender. May be served with rice.

Oriental Chicken

3 chicken breasts, halved, skinned, boned and cut into strips
¼ cup lite sodium soy sauce
1 onion, sliced
2 celery stalks, sliced diagonally
2 carrots, chopped
6 mushrooms, sliced

1 cup fresh snow peas or 1 (10–ounce) package frozen
3 tablespoons Fleischmann's Fat Free Squeezable Spread
¾ cup chicken broth
2 tablespoons lite sodium soy sauce
1 tablespoon cornstarch
Salt and pepper to taste
½ cup alfalfa sprouts

Marinate chicken in ¼ cup soy sauce for 1 hour and drain. Sauté first 5 vegetables in Pam–sprayed, non–stick skillet for 2 minutes. Vegetables must stay crisp. Cook chicken strips in Pam–sprayed skillet until chicken turns white. Make sauce out of Fleischmann's, broth, 2 tablespoons soy sauce, cornstarch, salt and pepper. Add sauce to chicken and vegetables and heat thoroughly for 3 minutes. Add sprouts. Serve on bed of rice.

Skillet Dinner

1 pound Country Turkey Sausage (see page 218)
½ cup onion, chopped
¼ cup green pepper, chopped
1 (16–ounce) can chopped tomatoes
1 cup elbow macaroni, uncooked

½ cup tomato juice (or water)
1 tablespoon sugar
1 teaspoon salt
½ teaspoon chili powder
1 cup fat–free sour cream
Pepper to taste

Cook sausage in colander in microwave. Meanwhile, sauté onions and pepper in a non–stick, Pam–sprayed skillet. Mix sausage, onion and peppers. Add tomatoes, macaroni, tomato juice, sugar and seasonings. Stir in sour cream. Heat thoroughly, but do not boil.

Chicken and Broccoli Rice Casserole

½ cup onions, diced
½ cup mushrooms, silced
2 cups rice, cooked and hot
2 cups chicken breasts, boned, skinned and cubed
2 cups broccoli, steamed

1 can Campbell's Healthy Request cream of mushroom soup
½ cup fat–free Cheddar cheese, shredded
1 tablespoon Fleischmann's Fat Free Squeezable Spread

In a Pam–sprayed non–stick skillet, sauté onions and mushrooms. Stir in remaining ingredients. Bake at 350° for 20 to 25 minutes.

Chicken Scampi

6 chicken breast halves, boned and skinned
2 tablespoons Ultra Promise 70% Less Fat
¼ cup Fleischmann's Fat Free Squeezable Spread

½ teaspoon minced garlic
⅛ cup fresh lemon juice
¼ cup dry white wine
1 tablespoon oregano
1 teaspoon basil
Rice

Cut chicken into bite–size pieces. Cook chicken and garlic in Pam–sprayed skillet until done. Add remaining ingredients and cook 15 to 20 minutes. Serve over rice.

Baked Halibut

2 teaspoons rosemary
½ teaspoon marjoram

1 cup Dijon mustard
Halibut fillets

Mix together first 3 ingredients. Brush on fillets. Let sit for 30 minutes, then bake at 350° for 30 minutes or until done.

NOTE: Trout may be used in place of halibut.

Baked Cream Fish

2 pounds fish fillets
1 can Healthy Choice cream of
  mushroom soup
½ cup skim milk
1 tablespoon dry mustard

½ cup bread crumbs
½ tablespoon parsley flakes
Paprika
Tarragon

Cut fish in serving–size pieces, about ¼ inch to ½ inch thick. Place in Pam–sprayed baking dish. Sprinkle with lemon juice. Combine soup, milk and mustard; pour over fish. Top with crumbs. Sprinkle with parsley. Generously sprinkle with tarragon. Bake at 350° for about 35 minutes or until done.

Baked Shrimp

2 tablespoons Ultra Promise
  70% Fat Free
6 tablespoons Fleischmann's
  Fat Free Squeezable Spread
2 pounds shrimp, peeled and
  uncooked
2 teaspoons tarragon

½ cup sherry
½ cup fresh parsley, chopped
3 to 4 cloves garlic, minced
½ teaspoon paprika
¼ teaspoon white pepper
2 cups fresh bread crumbs

Combine ingredients in shallow baking dish. Cover and bake at 350° for 30 minutes.

Broiled Orange Roughy

Orange roughy fillets
Lemon pepper

Paprika
Rice, cooked

Sprinkle fillets with lemon pepper and paprika on both sides. Broil 7 to 9 minutes or until crisp and fish flakes with a fork. Serve with rice.

Baked Stuffed Flounder

½ cup celery, finely chopped
½ cup green onions, sliced
1 clove garlic, minced
1½ cups bread crumbs
3 tablespoons mustard, prepared
2 tablespoons Weight Watcher's Fat Free Whipped Dressing
½ pound boiled shrimp, chopped
½ pound Louis Rich imitation crabmeat
1 Egg Beater
1 tablespoon lemon juice
¼ cup Fleischmann's Fat Free Squeezable Spread
Salt, black pepper and cayenne pepper to taste
4 medium–size flounder
I Can't Believe It's Not Butter spray

Sauté celery, onions and garlic in non–stick, Pam–sprayed skillet. Add remaining ingredients except shrimp and crab; mix well. Add seafood. Split thick side of flounder, lengthwise and crosswise, and loosen meat from bone to form pocket. Spray pocket with I Can't Believe It's Not Butter spray and stuff. Place fish in a Pam–sprayed shallow baking dish; do not overlap. Brush with Fleischmann's. Cover and bake at 375° for 25 minutes or until fish flakes with a fork. Remove cover and bake another 5 minutes.

Crab Cakes

2 (6½–ounce) cans crabmeat
¼ cup onion, finely diced
1 cup bread crumbs
2 Egg Beaters
2 teaspoons prepared mustard
⅛ teaspoon Cayenne pepper
Salt and pepper to taste
I Can't Believe It's Not Butter spray

Combine all ingredients; cover. Refrigerate at least 30 minutes to allow flavors to blend. (This may be made up several hours before cooking). Shape into patties. Spray a non–stick skillet with Pam and "fry" until golden. Spray each patty with Pam and turn over immediately and cook until golden. Spray each patty with butter spray and cook 1 minute longer on each side. Serve hot.

Crunchy Tuna Casserole

1 cup rice
1 (6–ounce) can water
  chestnuts, drained and
  chopped
¼ cup celery, finely chopped
½ cup green pepper, finely
  chopped
1 can Healthy Request cream of
  mushroom soup

2 tablespoons fresh lemon
  juice
Salt to taste
1 teaspoon Worcestershire
  sauce
1 teaspoon soy sauce
1 (7–ounce) can water–packed
  tuna, drained
6 fat–free saltines, crumbled

Cook rice according to directions. Combine all ingredients except tuna and saltines. Stir in tuna. Pour into a Pam–sprayed casserole dish. Cover. Bake at 350° for 25 minutes. Uncover. Add crumbled saltines and bake, uncovered for an additional 5 minutes.

Easy Sole Fillets

3 pounds sole fillets
1 cup Weight Watcher's Fat
  Free Whipped Dressing
1 teaspoon tarragon

1 cup fat–free Parmesan cheese
1 cup bread crumbs
  (see page 161)
1 teaspoon paprika

In a Pam–sprayed baking dish, place fillets. Spread with whipped dressing. Combine tarragon, cheese, bread crumbs and paprika. Sprinkle over fish. Bake at 350° for 30 minutes.

Flounder Dijon

1½ pounds flounder fillets
Freshly ground black pepper
Dijon mustard

½ cup white wine
1 lemon cut in wedges

Rinse and dry fillets. Pepper on both sides. Lightly coat with mustard. Lightly brown fillets in a non–stick, Pam–sprayed skillet. Add wine; cover; simmer 3–5 minutes. Serve with lemon wedges.

One Pan Meal

1 box low-fat macaroni and
  cheese
¼ cup Fleischmann's Fat Free
  Squeezable Spread
½ cup skim milk, divided
1 (8½-ounce) can green peas

1 (6½-ounce) can water packed
  tuna, drained
1 can Campbell's Healthy
  Request cream of mushroom
  soup

Cook macaroni noodles in salted water. Drain. Add Fleischmann's,
¼ cup skim milk and cheese sauce mix; mix well. Add remaining
ingredients. Bake at 350° for 30 minutes or until thoroughly heated.

Oven-Fried Fish

2 pounds fish fillets
½ cup skim milk
1 cup bread crumbs

McCormick Parsley Patch salt
  free lemon pepper
I Can't Believe It's Not Butter
  spray

Cut fillets into serving-size portions. Dip fish into milk and roll into
crumbs. Liberally sprinkle with lemon pepper and spray with butter
spray. Place onto a Pam-sprayed baking dish. Place pan on shelf
near top of oven and bake at 500° 10 to 20 minutes. Watch carefully as
fish cooks. Serve immediately.

Tuna Noodle Casserole

2 cups No Yolk egg noodles,
  cooked
1 (6½-ounce) can water-packed
  tuna, drained
1 (16-ounce) can peas and
  carrots, drained

1 can Campbell's Healthy
  Request cream of mushroom
  soup
¼ cup evaporated skimmed milk
½ cup fat-free Cheddar cheese,
  shredded

Mix together all ingredients, excluding the noodles, mixing well.
Fold in noodles. Place in a Pam-sprayed casserole dish. Bake at 350°
for 25 minutes or until bubbly.

Grilled Salmon

2 teaspoons lemon zest, grated
2 teaspoons lime zest, grated
1 tablespoon garlic, minced
Salt and pepper to taste
1 tablespoon fresh parsley,
  chopped
1 tablespoon fresh thyme,
  chopped
Weight Watcher's Fat Free
  Whipped Dressing
4 salmon steaks

Combine first 6 ingredients; set aside. Lightly brush steaks with whipped dressing; sprinkle with herb mixture. Place salmon under hot broiler; cook for 3 minutes. Turn; broil an additional 3 minutes. Salmon should appear opaque at its center when done.

Imperial Salmon

1 (16–ounce) can salmon,
  drained and deboned
½ cup green pepper, finely
  chopped
½ cup onion, finely chopped
3 tablespoons Fleischmann's
  Fat Free Squeezable Spread
1 tablespoon Ultra Promise
  70% Fat Free
¼ cup flour
1½ cups skim milk
Salt and pepper to taste
2 tablespoons pimento,
  chopped
1 teaspoon prepared mustard
Tabasco to taste
1 (8½–ounce) can peas and
  carrots, cooked and drained
Low fat biscuits, cornbread or
  toast

Sauté onions and peppers in a non–stick, Pam–sprayed skillet. Make a paste with Fleischmann's, Promise, flour and a small amount of milk. Whisk remainder of milk into a paste. Cook over low heat, whisking constantly to remove all lumps. Cook until thick. Add salt and pepper. Add peas and carrots, pimento, mustard and Tabasco. Add salmon. Serve over bread of your choice.

Salmon Croquettes

2 (6–ounce) cans Chicken of
the Sea (2 fat grams per
serving) salmon
2 tablespoons onion, extra
finely chopped
2 tablespoons green pepper,
extra finely chopped

¾ cup cornmeal
¼ cup flour
1 Egg Beater
½ teaspoon lemon pepper
Salt and pepper to taste

Mix together salmon, onion, green pepper, lemon pepper and Egg Beater. Add cornmeal and flour gradually. Add salt and pepper. Preheat a non–stick skillet and spray with Pam. "Fry" salmon patties, turning once. Spray patties with Pam spray before turning. Cook until done. Makes 6 croquettes.

Salmon Surprise Patties

1 (1–pound) can salmon
½ cup Whipped Potatoes
(see page 271)
¼ cup celery, thinly sliced
3 tablespoons onions, finely
chopped
1 Egg Beater

1 teaspoon Worcestershire
sauce
¼ teaspoon salt
Pepper to taste
½ cup bread crumbs
Fat–free Cheddar cheese slices
1 cup cornflake crumbs

Drain salmon. Remove bones and skin; flake with fork. Combine salmon with next 8 ingredients; mix well. Pat out an even number of patties. Cut cheese slightly smaller than patties. Place cheese on top of ½ of the patties. Cover with remaining patties, making sure edges are sealed. Roll in cornflake crumbs. Spray a non–stick skillet with Pam. Cook over medium heat until golden. Spray each patty with Pam and turn immediately and cook to golden. Serve hot.

VARIATION: For added zip, sprinkle patty liberally with lemon pepper seasoning before adding cheese. Continue with directions.

Scallops au Gratin

1 package Louis Rich imitation
  scallops
⅛ cup onion, chopped
¼ cup celery, chopped
¼ cup green pepper, chopped
2 tablespoons Ultra Promise
  70% Less Fat
⅛ cup flour

¼ cup skim milk
¼ cup evaporated skimmed
  milk
Salt and pepper to taste
2 cups rice, cooked
5 slices fat–free American
  cheese

Sauté onion, celery and pepper in a non–stick, Pam–sprayed skillet. Make a paste with Promise and flour. Gradually add skim milk, whisking to remove lumps. Add evaporated skimmed milk. Cook over medium heat, stirring constantly. Cook until thick. Add onion mixture and scallops. Place rice in the bottom of a Pam–sprayed casserole dish. Add three slices of cheese on top of rice. Add scallop mixture. Bake, covered, at 350° for 20 minutes. Remove from oven and place remaining cheese on top. Return to oven, uncovered, and cook an additional 7 to 10 minutes. Serve hot.

Seafood Lasagna

6 lasagna noodles, cooked
  according to package
  directions
1 cup onions, diced
2 cups fat–free mozzarella
  cheese, shredded
2½ cups fat–free cottage cheese
1½ cups fat–free ricotta cheese
3 Egg Beaters

2 teaspoons basil
¼ teaspoon pepper
2 cans Campbell's Healthy
  Request cream of mushroom
  soup
¼ cup evaporated skimmed
  milk
Butter salt
Fat–free Parmesan cheese

Sauté onions in a Pam–sprayed, non–stick skillet. Add cheeses, Egg Beaters, basil and pepper. In a separate bowl, combine soup, milk and wine; add crabmeat. In a 9 x 13–inch Pam–sprayed casserole dish, layer 3 noodles to cover bottom. Arrange half of shrimp on top of noodles. Add half of cheese on top of shrimp. Spread half of soup mixture on cheese. Sprinkle with butter salt. Repeat. Sprinkle top with fat–free Parmesan cheese. Bake at 350° for 45 minutes or until bubbly.

Shrimp Soufflé

1 pound medium shrimp,
   peeled and deveined
6 slices fat–free bread, cut into
   bite–size pieces
3 ounces Kroger Lite Classics
   sharp Cheddar cheese,
   shredded
5 ounces fat–free Cheddar
   cheese, shredded

2 tablespoons Ultra Promise
   70% Less Fat
2 tablespoons Fleischmann's
   Fat Free Squeezable Spread
3 Egg Beaters
½ teaspoon dry mustard
¼ cup white wine
2 cups skim milk

Place prepared bread into a Pam–sprayed baking dish. Top with shrimp and cheeses. Combine remaining ingredients and pour over all. Cover and refrigerate overnight. Bake at 350°, covered, for one hour.

Spicy Shrimp and Rice

1 (10–ounce) bag frozen,
   cooked shrimp, thawed
2 cups rice, cooked
½ cup barbecue sauce

1 teaspoon vinegar
1 cup pineapple chunks,
   drained

Combine barbecue sauce and vinegar in saucepan. Add shrimp and rice. Cover and heat thoroughly. Stir in pineapple and serve.

Carolyn's Cheese Soufflé

5 slices white bread, trimmed
   and cubed
1 cup fat–free Cheddar cheese,
   shredded
4 Egg Beaters

2½ cups skim milk
1 teaspoon salt
1 teaspoon dry mustard
¼ teaspoon Tabasco sauce

Put cubed bread in a deep–dish Pam–sprayed casserole. Spread cheese over bread. Mix together remaining ingredients; pour over cheese. Refrigerate overnight. Bake at 350° for 40 minutes.

Company Sandwich

1 (8–ounce) package fat–free
  cream cheese
1 teaspoon (or to taste) garlic
  powder
1½ teaspoons dried chives
2 tablespoons green pepper,
  finely diced
2 tablespoons onion, finely
  diced
Fresh basil leaves

1 pound Healthy Choice Honey
  Ham
1 pound Healthy Choice Cajun
  roast beef
1½ cups fat–free mozzarella
  cheese, shredded
1½ cups fat–free Cheddar
  cheese, shredded
1 loaf French bread, cut
  lengthwise

Mix first 5 ingredients well. Cut bread in half lengthwise and spread cream cheese mixture on inside of bread halves. On bottom half of bread, layer basil leaves on top of cream cheese mixture. Layer half of the ham, followed by 1 cup of shredded cheeses. Layer remaining ham; then another cup of shredded cheeses. Layer half of the roast beef, followed by shredded cheeses and add remaining roast beef. Top with top half of French bread. Put sandwich back into the bag from which the bread came. Seal. Place in refrigerator. Place weights (two 5–pound bags of flour, etc.) on top of sandwich so it appears mashed. Leave overnight. When ready to serve, cut sandwiches into desired thicknesses.

Darrell's Scrambled Eggs

4 Egg Beaters
Lawry's season salt to taste

Tabasco sauce to taste

Mix together and pour into a non–stick, Pam–sprayed skillet. Cook over medium heat, stirring until done.

VARIATION: Stir in 2 slices Borden's fat–free American or sharp Cheddar cheese slices, chopped.

Garden Brunch Pie

1 (10–ounce) package frozen
chopped broccoli, cooked and
well drained
1 cup fat–free sour cream
1 cup fat–free cottage cheese,
drained
½ cup lowfat Pioneer biscuit
baking mix

¼ cup Ultra Promise 70% Less
Fat
2 Egg Beaters
1 tomato, peeled and thinly
sliced
¼ cup fat–free Parmesan cheese

Pam–spray a deep dish 9–inch pie plate. Spread broccoli in bottom of
plate. Beat sour cream, cottage cheese, baking mix, Promise and Egg
Beaters until smooth. Pour into plate. Arrange tomato slices on top.
Sprinkle with Parmesan cheese.

VARIATIONS: Substitute spinach in place of broccoli.

Layered Vegetable Sandwich

Foccacia bread
Hot salsa
Chavrie goat cheese (3 fat
grams per serving)
Roasted red pimento, whole

Red cabbage, thinly shredded
Tomato, thinly sliced
Red onion, cut in rings
Mushrooms, sliced
Fresh basil leaves

Cut bread lengthwise to fill sandwich. Layer sandwich in order
given, ending and beginning with bread.

Texas Skillet Dinner

1 box low–fat macaroni and
cheese
¼ cup Fleischmann's Fat Free
Squeezable Spread

¼ cup skim milk
1 (15–ounce) can chili beans
1½ tablespoons jalapeño
pepper relish

Cook macaroni noodles in salted water. Drain. Add Fleischmann's,
milk and cheese sauce mix; mix well. Add remaining ingredients.
Bake at 350° for 30 minutes or until thoroughly heated.

Turkey Cranberry Sandwiches

Turkey slices
1 can whole cranberry sauce,
   chilled
Lettuce leaves

Weight Watcher's Fat Free
   Whipped Dressing (optional)
Whole wheat bread

Spread bread with whipped dressing; add turkey slices. Top turkey with a thin slice of cranberry sauce. Add lettuce. Top with second slice of bread.

Apricot–Mustard Pork

½ cup apricot preserves
½ cup Griffin's sweet mustard

1½ pounds Bryan's pork
   tenderloin
Salt and pepper to taste

Salt and pepper tenderloin and place in a Pam–sprayed casserole dish. In a small bowl, combine preserves and mustard. Pour this mixture over tenderloin. Cover. Bake at 350° for 10 minutes. Uncover and bake an additional 35 to 40 minutes or until done.

Baked Ham Omelette

¼ cup flour
1 teaspoon baking powder
12 Egg Beaters
5 drops Tabasco
Salt and pepper to taste

2¼ cups fat–free mozzarella
   cheese, shredded
2 cups turkey ham, finely
   chopped
2½ tablespoons Ultra Promise
   70% Less Fat, melted

Sift flour and baking powder into a 9 x 13–inch baking dish. Beat Egg Beaters, Tabasco, salt and pepper. Add cheese and turkey ham. Pour into baking dish. Pour Ultra Promise over all. Bake at 400° for 15 minutes; reduce heat to 350° and bake 10 to 15 minutes longer. Cut into squares.

Bacon Fettuccine

1 Egg Beater
2 tablespoons evaporated
  skimmed milk
4 ounces fettuccine
2 teaspoons Ultra Promise 70%
  Less Fat
¼ cup fat–free grated Parmesan
  cheese

1 tablespoon dried parsley
1 piece Oscar Mayer bacon,
  fried crisp, drained
Dash of salt
Garlic powder to taste
Coarsely ground black pepper

In a small mixing bowl stir together the Egg Beater, milk, salt, pepper, and garlic; set aside. In a large saucepan, cook fettuccine according to package directions, except omitting the oil and salt. Drain well. Return pasta to hot saucepan. Immediately pour the egg mixture over pasta. Add Promise. Heat and stir mixture over low heat until thickens and pasta is well coated. Add Parmesan cheese, parsley and cooked bacon pieces; toss until combined. Serve immediately.

Baked Pork Chops and Rice

¾ cup uncooked rice
4 center cut pork chops, well
  trimmed
1 onion, sliced
1½ cups apricot nectar

⅓ cup brown sugar
1 teaspoon dry mustard
¼ teaspoon salt
¼ teaspoon pepper
1 teaspoon Ultra Promise 70%
  Less Fat

Place rice in a Pam–sprayed baking dish. Arrange chops on top. Add onion slices. Combine remaining ingredients and pour over all. Cover and bake at 350° for 1 hour.

Baked Pork Tenderloin

1 Bryan tenderloin
Salt to taste
Pepper to taste

Sherry Wine Sauce
(see page 82)

Season tenderloin with salt and pepper. Place on a foil–lined Pam–sprayed cooking sheet. Bake at 350° for 45 minutes. Serve with Sherry Wine Sauce.

Barbecued Tenderloin

1 Bryan tenderloin

1 envelope Shake–N–Bake barbecue for chicken or pork

Roll tenderloin in Shake–N–Bake. Place on a foil–lined Pam–sprayed cooking sheet. Bake at 350° for 45 minutes.

Broccoli & Ham Strata

6 slices whole wheat bread,
  edges removed and cubed
2 cups skim milk
3 tablespoons mustard
4 Egg Beaters

Salt and pepper to taste
1 (10–ounce) package frozen
  broccoli
1 cup turkey ham, diced

Cook broccoli according to package directions; drain well and set aside. Place prepared bread in a 2–quart Pam–sprayed casserole dish. Layer broccoli and ham on top of bread. Combine remaining ingredients and pour over broccoli and ham. Cover. Refrigerate overnight. Next morning uncover and bake at 350° for 40 minutes or until knife inserted in middle comes out clean.

Cherry Pork Chops

1½ pounds tenderloin
1 teaspoon salt
¼ teaspoon pepper
1 (1–pound) can tart, red
   cherries

1 tablespoon + 1 teaspoon
   cornstarch
¼ cup brown sugar

Sprinkle tenderloin with salt and pepper. Bake at 425° for 20 minutes. Drain cherries, reserving juice and adding enough water to make 1 cup liquid. Combine cornstarch and sugar. Cook, stirring constantly until thickened and clear. Add cherries to sauce. Pour over tenderloin. Cover tightly and bake at 350° for 45 minutes.

Country Turkey Sausage

1 pound extra lean ground
   turkey
1 tablespoon rubbed sage

½ teaspoon crushed red pepper
½ teaspoon salt
⅛ teaspoon black pepper

Mix well. Store in refrigerator until needed for cooking. Keeps up to one week.

Curried Pork Tenderloin with Cranberries

4 teaspoons curry powder
½ teaspoon ginger (powdered)
1½ pounds Bryan pork
   tenderloin

½ teaspoon salt
½ teaspoon pepper
1 can whole cranberry sauce
¼ cup dry white wine

Combine curry and ginger. Rub mixture into tenderloin. In a small mixing bowl, combine salt, pepper, cranberry sauce and wine. Heat, stirring until simmering. Place tenderloin in a Pam–sprayed casserole dish. Bake in a 350° oven for 15 minutes. Remove tenderloin from oven and pour sauce over tenderloin. Return to oven and cook uncovered for about 45 minutes or until meat is done and tender.

Farmer Pork Chops

¾ pound tenderloin
Garlic powder
Salt to taste
Pepper to taste
4 cups Irish potatoes, peeled,
   sliced and cooked until
   tender crisp and cooled

1 large onion, sliced
1½ cups fat–free sour cream
2 teaspoons mustard
1½ teaspoons Lawry's seasoned
   salt
¼ teaspoon garlic powder

Preheat oven to 425°. Sprinkle tenderloin with salt, pepper and garlic powder. Cook, uncovered for 20 minutes or until almost done. Mix together sour cream, mustard, seasoned salt and garlic powder. Sauté onions in a Pam–sprayed non–stick skillet. Mix together potatoes, onions and sour cream mixture. Bake at 350° for 30 minutes. Slice cooked tenderloin and place on top of potato mixture. Bake an additional 15 minutes or until bubbly.

Ham & Broccoli Skillet Supper

3½ cups water
1 package Kroger au gratin
   potato mix
2 cups fresh broccoli, chopped
¼ cup onion, chopped
1 tablespoon Ultra Promise
   70% Less Fat

3 tablespoons Fleischmann's
   Fat Free Squeezable Spread
1 cup diced turkey ham
½ cup skim milk
1 dash Lawry's seasoned salt
⅛ teaspoon black pepper
3 drops Tabasco (optional)
5 Egg Beaters

In a skillet, bring water to a boil; add potato slices. Reduce heat; cover and let simmer 10 minutes. Add broccoli; cover and let simmer 5 minutes; drain. Sauté onion in a Pam–sprayed non–stick skillet. Stir in onion, Ultra Promise, Fleischmann's and turkey ham. In a small bowl, combine contents of seasoning mix, milk, Lawry's, pepper and Tabasco; stir until smooth. Add Egg Beaters and mix well. Pour over potato mixture in skillet. Cover; cook over low heat 20 to 30 minutes or until eggs are set.

NOTE: Best if done in a non–stick skillet.

Ham Strata

2 cups low fat or fat–free ham, chopped
6 slices fat–free wheat bread, crust removed and cubed
5 Egg Beaters
2 cups skim milk
1½ cups fat–free Cheddar cheese, shredded
1 teaspoon salt
1 teaspoon dry mustard
2 tablespoons prepared mustard

Layer bread cubes, ham and cheese in a Pam–sprayed 9 x 13–inch casserole dish. Mix remaining ingredients and pour over top. Refrigerate overnight. Bake, uncovered, at 350° for 45 minutes or until a knife inserted in the middle comes out clean.

Ina's Pork Platter with Horseradish Sauce

1 (12–ounce) can beer
2 tablespoons Worcestershire sauce
1 tablespoon minced onion
2 teaspoons prepared mustard
½ teaspoon salt
Pepper to taste
2 tablespoons brown sugar
1 (3–pound) pork tenderloin

Combine first 7 ingredients and mix well. Place tenderloin and marinade in glass or plastic dish and marinate overnight in refrigerator. Roast at 350° for 1 hour or until well done. Serve with Horseradish Sauce.

HORSERADISH SAUCE:
⅔ cup fat–free sour cream
2 tablespoons prepared horseradish

Combine and serve with pork.

Louisiana Sausage & Rice

½ small onion, diced
2½ cups water
4 beef bouillon cubes
Few drops of Tabasco

¼ teaspoon oregano
1 teaspoon dry minced onion
1 cup dry rice
1 pound Bryan Light sausage

Sauté onion in a non–stick Pam–sprayed skillet. Add bouillon, water and seasonings. Heat to boiling. In a Pam–sprayed casserole dish add dry rice and hot liquid. Bake at 350°, covered, for 50 minutes. Meanwhile, cook sausage in a colander in a microwave so fat drippings will cook out. Add to casserole. Heat, uncovered, for 10 minutes.

Mardi Gras Surprise

1 pound red beans, dried
1 package Butterball Fat Free
  smoked turkey sausage,
  diced
⅔ cup celery, diced
1 onion, chopped

1 garlic clove, crushed
1 teaspoon sugar
Salt to taste
1 bay leaf
8 to 10 cups water
1½ cups white rice, uncooked

Rinse beans. In a large pot combine beans, celery, onion, garlic, sugar, salt, bay leaf and water. Cook until done, stirring occasionally. Add uncooked rice and sausage and cook until done, about 15 to 20 minutes longer. Serve hot.

Orange Baked Pork

1½ pounds Bryan pork
  tenderloin
½ cup orange juice
1 teaspoon salt
¼ teaspoon pepper

½ teaspoon ground mustard
¼ cup brown sugar
2 tablespoons orange
  marmalade

Combine all ingredients excluding tenderloin. Place tenderloin in a Pam–sprayed casserole dish. Pour orange juice mixture over all. Bake at 350° for 45 to 50 minutes or until done. Baste occasionally during cooking.

Marilyn's Ham & Asparagus Strata

6 slices whole wheat bread,
    edges removed and cubed
2 cups skim milk
4 Egg Beaters
3 tablespoons mustard
Salt and pepper to taste

1 (14.5–ounce) can asparagus,
    drained
1 cup turkey ham, diced
1 can Healthy Choice cream of
    mushroom soup
½ cup skim milk

Place prepared bread in a 2–quart Pam–sprayed casserole dish. Combine milk, Egg Beaters, mustard, salt and pepper. Pour this mixture over bread. Arrange asparagus and ham on top. Cover and refrigerate overnight. The next morning combine soup and ½ cup milk. Pour this on top of entire casserole. Bake covered at 350° for 45 minutes; uncovered and bake an additional 15 minutes. Serve hot.

Pork Chops & Apricots in Curry Sauce

1½ pounds pork tenderloin
Salt to taste
Pepper to taste
1 (8–ounce) can apricots
1 (5–ounce) can mushrooms
1 medium onion, sliced

2 tablespoons Fleischmann's
    Fat Free Squeezable Spread
1 can Campbell's Healthy
    Request cream of mushroom
    soup
¼ cup dry white wine
½ tablespoon curry powder

Place tenderloin in a Pam–sprayed pan. Sprinkle with salt and pepper. Drain apricots reserving ¼ cup juice. Place apricots on top of tenderloin. Sauté mushrooms and onions in a Pam–sprayed non-stick skillet. Top tenderloin with onion mixture. In a small bowl, combine remaining ingredients. Pour this over meat. Bake, uncovered, at 350° for 1 hour. May be served over rice.

Pork Chop Bake

1 pound carrots, pared and
   sliced
2 onions, sliced thinly
8 center cut pork chops
2 teaspoons sage

Salt and pepper to taste
3 tart apples, pared and
   quartered
¼ cup brown sugar

Place carrots in the bottom of a Pam–sprayed shallow casserole dish.
Top with onions. Overlap chops and sprinkle with sage, salt and
pepper. Add apples and sprinkle with brown sugar. Cover and bake
at 350° for 2½ hours. Uncover and bake another 30 minutes.

Pork Chops Dijon

4 pork loin chops
1 medium onion
3 tablespoons Dijon mustard
2 tablespoons fat–free Italian
   salad dressing

1 teaspoon Weight Watcher's
   Fat Free Whipped Dressing
¼ teaspoon pepper

Pam–spray a non–stick skillet. Brown chops on both sides. Remove
chops; add onions. Cook until transparent. Combine mustard, dressing, whipped dressing and pepper. Brush over chops. Cover and
cook an additional 10 to 15 minutes.

Pork Tenderloin Casserole

6 center cut pork chops
4 cups bread crumbs, corn
  bread and light bread, mixed
½ cup celery, chopped
½ cup onion, chopped
Poultry seasoning to taste

1 can chicken broth
1 can Campbell's Healthy
  Request cream of celery soup
¾ cup evaporated skimmed
  milk
Salt and pepper to taste

Salt and pepper pork chops and brown in a non–stick Pam–sprayed skillet. Set aside. Sauté celery and onion in same Pam–sprayed skillet. Add bread crumbs and enough broth to make the desired consistency. Add poultry seasoning. Pour into a Pam–sprayed casserole dish. Place pork chops on top. Mix together soup and milk. Pour over top of chops. Bake at 350° for 30 minutes or until thoroughly heated.

Pork Tenderloin with Onion Gravy

1 (3– to 4–pound) pork
  tenderloin
1 envelope Lipton onion soup

½ cup water
¼ cup flour

Place a sheet of aluminum foil in a baking pan. Sprinkle with onion soup. Roll tenderloin in soup mix. Fold foil over meat and seal securely. Cook at 350° for approximately 3 hours or until well done.

Open foil and remove meat but keep it warm. Measure drippings and enough water to make 2 cups. Pour this into pan. Mix the ½ cup water with the flour and add this to the pan. Heat to boiling, stirring constantly. Boil until desired thickness. Add meat to gravy. Serve hot.

Quick Sweet and Sour Pork

1½ pounds pork tenderloin,
  cut into strips
2 tablespoons Fleischmann's
  Fat Free Squeezable Spread
¼ cup water
½ teaspoon salt

½ medium green pepper
1 cup pineapple preserves
2 tablespoons vinegar
1 tablespoon soy sauce
¼ cup thinly sliced onion
Dash garlic

Brown pork in Pam–sprayed non–stick skillet. Add water and salt and simmer until tender, about 15 minutes; drain. Combine preserves, Fleischmann's, vinegar and soy sauce. Pour over tenderloin. Add remaining ingredients. Cook until thoroughly heated. Serve over rice.

Sandra's Bacon Quiche

8 slices Kraft fat–free Swiss
  cheese, diced
8 slices Jennie–O turkey bacon,
  cooked and crumbled
3 Egg Beaters
1 cup evaporated skimmed
  milk

½ cup skim milk
½ teaspoon salt
¼ teaspoon pepper
Dash cayenne pepper
½ teaspoon dry mustard
1 Pie Shell, unbaked
  (see page 327)

Place cheese and bacon in the bottom of pie shell. Beat together remaining ingredients and pour into pie shell. Bake at 375° for 35 minutes or until a knife inserted in the middle comes out clean.

Sausage and Rice Casserole

2 pounds Country Turkey
  Sausage (see page 218)
1 onion, finely chopped
¼ cup bell pepper, chopped
1 pound fresh mushrooms,
  sliced

2 cans Campbell's Healthy
  Request cream of chicken
  soup
1 cup fat–free sour cream
3 cups cooked rice

Cook sausage in colander in microwave so that fat can drain out. Cook until done. Sauté onion, pepper and mushrooms in Pam–sprayed non–stick skillet. Add to sausage mixture. Add soup and sour cream. Combine with rice. Pour into Pam–sprayed casserole. Bake at 350° for 45 minutes.

Sausage Apple Ring

¾ pound Bryan light pork
  sausage
1 cup fat–free cracker crumbs
2 Egg Beaters
¼ cup skim milk

¼ cup minced onion
1 cup finely chopped apples
½ teaspoon sugar
Egg Beaters, scrambled

Combine first 7 ingredients. Mix well. Press lightly into a wax lined 6–cup ring mold to shape. Turn out on shallow non–stick baking pan. Bake 30 minutes. Drain any excess fat from pan and continue baking for an additional 30 minutes. To serve, fill center of ring with scrambled Egg Beaters.

Sausage Cheese Strata

6 slices whole wheat bread,
  edges removed and diced
2 cups skim milk
4 Egg Beaters
3 tablespoons mustard
Salt and pepper to taste

1 pound Bryan Lite pork
  sausage
1¼ cups fat–free Cheddar
  cheese, shredded
1 can Healthy Choice cream of
  mushroom soup
½ cup skim milk

Cook sausage in colander in microwave oven. Set aside. Place prepared bread into a 2–quart Pam–sprayed casserole dish. Combine milk, Egg Beaters, mustard, salt and pepper. Pour over bread. Arrange sausage and cheese over top. Cover and refrigerate overnight. The next morning, combine soup and ½ cup milk. Pour over entire casserole. Cover and bake at 350° for 40 minutes. Uncover and bake an additional 20 minutes. Serve hot.

Sausage Rice Stuffing

1¼ cups uncooked wild rice
1¼ cups uncooked long grain
  rice
1 pound Country Turkey
  Sausage (see page 218)
4 ribs celery, diced

6 ounces fresh mushrooms,
  sliced
1 large onion, diced
Salt and pepper to taste
1 tablespoon Fleischmann's Fat
  Free Squeezable Spread

Prepare rice as directed. Toss together. Cook sausage in colander in microwave so any fat can cook out; add to rice. In a Pam–sprayed non–stick skillet, sauté celery, mushrooms and onion. Add to rice. Add salt, pepper and Fleischmann's. Mix well.

May be used for pork, poultry, etc. Or may be served as main dish.

Smoked Sausage and Sauerkraut

1 (14–ounce) Butterball Fat Free
    smoked turkey sausage,
    diced
1 can Bavarian style sauerkraut
1 cup water

1 potato, peeled and grated
1 carrot, peeled and grated
⅛ teaspoon black pepper
1 onion, chopped

In a Pam–sprayed non–stick skillet sauté onions until done. Add sauerkraut and cook for 2 minutes. Add water and sausage; cook 15 minutes. Add potato, carrot, and pepper. Cook 5 additional minutes.

Vegetable Pork Chop Dinner

4 (½–inch) center cut pork
    chops
½ teaspoon salt
¼ teaspoon pepper
1 bay leaf
1½ cups V–8 juice

½ cup water
½ large head cabbage, cut in
    wedges
3 carrots, sliced
1 cup onion, chopped
4 small new potatoes, halved

Sprinkle chops with salt and pepper. Brown in a non–stick Pam–sprayed skillet. Remove chops to a casserole dish. Add bay leaf and V–8 juice; cover and bake at 350° for 30 minutes. Add remaining ingredients; cover and continue baking 35 to 40 minutes or until vegetables are tender. Remove bay leaf before serving.

Beef Burgundy

2 pounds beef tenderloin	Salt to taste
2 medium onions, sliced	Pepper to taste
1 teaspoon garlic powder	¼ teaspoon thyme
3 tablespoons Fleischmann's	¼ teaspoon marjoram
Fat Free Squeezable Spread	¼ teaspoon oregano
2 cans beef gravy	1 small can mushrooms
½ cup Burgundy	

Cut meat into cubes. Sauté onions in Pam–sprayed non–stick skillet. Remove onions and brown meat sprinkled with garlic. Add gravy, wine and spices. Add onions and drained mushrooms. Simmer, covered, for 2 hours or until tender. Serve over rice or noodles.

Beef Biscuit Roll–ups

1 pound ground round	¾ teaspoon salt
½ cup onion, chopped fine	⅛ teaspoon pepper
2 tablespoons green pepper, chopped fine	¼ teaspoon celery salt
	1 Egg Beater
2 tablespoons Weight Watcher's Fat Free Whipped Dressing	3¼ cups Pioneer Low–fat Biscuit mix
	1 cup skim milk
2 tablespoon ketchup	

Cook ground round in colander in microwave so that fat can drain out. Cook until done. Sauté onions and peppers in Pam–sprayed non–stick skillet. Add to beef mixture. Add whipped dressing, ketchup, salt, pepper, celery salt and Egg Beater. Set aside. Prepare biscuit mix and milk. Turn out on lightly floured board. Roll into 12 x 18–inch rectangle. Spread meat mixture evenly over surface. Roll as for jelly roll. Cut into 12 slices about 1½–inch thick. Place into Pam–sprayed baking pan. Bake at 425° for 25 minutes.

VARIATION: Mix 1 envelope taco seasoning mix to cooked meat mixture.

Beef Niçoise

1½ pounds beef top round
  steak
1½ cups water
1½ beef bouillon
2 large onions
2½ teaspoons garlic powder
2 large tomatoes, peeled and
  diced
3 tablespoons capers

½ cup tomato puree
½ cup low fat beef gravy
1 teaspoon basil
¼ teaspoon oregano
1 teaspoon sugar
Salt to taste
Pepper to taste
½ cup chopped parsley

Pound round steak so to tenderize it. Cut into bite–sized pieces. Add water and bouillon and cook slowly until meat is tender and well done; drain and set aside. Sauté onions in a Pam–sprayed non–stick skillet. Add garlic, tomatoes, and capers. When mixture begins to cook, add puree, gravy, seasonings and parsley. Add meat and cook until slightly thick. May be served with rice.

Beef Stroganoff

3 cups beef tenderloin, diced
1 bay leaf
1 teaspoon salt
⅛ teaspoon pepper
1 envelope Lipton onion soup

1 can Campbell's Healthy
  Request cream of mushroom
  soup
1 (4–ounce) can sliced
  mushrooms, drained
⅓ cup red wine
Cooked rice

In a medium saucepan add meat, bay leaf, salt and pepper and enough water to cover meat. Cover, bring to a boil, reduce heat and simmer until tender. Drain cooked meat. Discard bay leaf. Add soup mix, soup, mushrooms and wine to meat mixture. Mix well. Spoon into lightly Pam–sprayed casserole dish. Bake at 350° for 30 minutes or until bubbly. Serve over rice or noodles.

Beef Tarragon

½ cup flour	1 cup beef broth
1½ teaspoons tarragon, divided	1 tablespoon sugar
1½ pounds beef tenderloin	5 ounces mushrooms
1 teaspoon garlic powder	1 bunch green onions, chopped
½ cup red wine vinegar	

Mix flour with 1 teaspoon tarragon; coat meat. In a Pam–sprayed non–stick skillet, cook meat just until browned. (Spray skillet before turning meat). Add garlic, vinegar, beef broth and sugar; cover and simmer for 1 hour and 15 minutes or until meat is tender. Check occasionally to see if more beef broth is needed. Sauté onions and mushrooms in another Pam–sprayed non–stick skillet. Add to meat mixture. Simmer an additional 10 minutes. Serve with noodles or rice.

Easy Beef Stroganoff

1 pound beef sirloin	1 tablespoon tomato paste
1 cup mushrooms, sliced	1¼ cups beef bouillon
½ cup onions, chopped	1 cup fat–free sour cream
1 clove garlic, minced	3 tablespoons sherry
2 tablespoons flour	

Have butcher slice beef sirloin into ¼–inch strips. In a Pam–sprayed skillet brown meat on bot sides; remove meat and discard drippings, if any. Pam–spray skillet again and add mushrooms, onions, and garlic and sauté. Remove vegetables. Mix together tomato paste and flour; add bouillon. Cook on medium–low heat until thick. Return meat and vegetables to pan with sauce in skillet; add sherry. Heat briefly. Remove from heat; add sour cream. Serve immediately. May be served over rice or eggless noodles.

Easy Spaghetti Casserole

½ pound Healthy Lean ground
  beef, cooked and drained
1 (25.75–ounce) jar Healthy
  Choice Super Chunky pasta
  sauce

½ pound spaghetti noodles,
  cooked and drained
1 cup fat–free Cheddar cheese,
  shredded
Parmesan cheese

In a Pam–sprayed cooking dish place half of noodles, half of cheese
and half of sauce. Make second layer of noodles, cheese and sauce.
Top with Parmesan cheese. Bake in 350° oven for 30 minutes or until
heated through.

Grandmother's Casserole

¾ pound ground round
1 cup onion, chopped
¼ cup green peppers, chopped
2 medium cans tomatoes
1 tablespoon ketchup
1 tablespoon Heinz 57 sauce
1½ cups cooked elbow or small
  seashell macaroni

Salt and pepper to taste
1 can Campbell's Healthy
  Request cream of mushroom
  soup
1 cup fat–free Cheddar cheese,
  shredded

Cook ground chuck in a colander in the microwave, stirring occasionally until done. In a Pam–sprayed non–stick skillet sauté onions
and pepper. Add tomatoes, ketchup, Heinz 57, salt and pepper.
Simmer for 3 minutes. Cook macaroni according to package directions. Combine macaroni, meat and cheese. Gently spoon meat mixture into soup. Pour into Pam–sprayed casserole dish. Bake at 350°
for 30 minutes.

Lasagna

12 lasagna noodles
¾ pound ground round
1 onion, chopped
1 green pepper, chopped
½ pound fat–free turkey
  smoked sausage, sliced
1 (4–ounce) can mushrooms,
  drained

4½ cups tomato sauce
½ pound fat–free ricotta cheese
½ pound fat–free mozzarella
  cheese
¼ cup fat–free Cheddar cheese,
  for topping

Cook noodles according to package directions, drain and set aside. Meanwhile, cook ground round in a colander in microwave until done. Sauté onions and green peppers in a non–stick Pam–sprayed skillet. Mix onions, peppers, ground round, sausage and mushrooms. In a 9 x 13–inch Pam–sprayed casserole dish, spread a thin layer of tomato sauce; add a layer of noodles, meat mixture and cheeses. Repeat layers ending with sauce and Cheddar cheese. Bake at 400° for 15 minutes or until bubbly. Let stand a few minutes before serving.

Manicotti

2 boxes manicotti shells
2 cups fat–free cottage cheese
2 cups fat–free mozzarella
  cheese, shredded
2 Egg Beaters

1 tablespoons parsley flakes
1 recipe Spaghetti Sauce
  (see page 81)
¼ cup fat–free Parmesan cheese

Cook manicotti according to package directions. Mix together cottage cheese, mozzarella cheese, Egg Beaters and parsley flakes. Stuff shells with cheese mixture. In a 9 x 13–inch Pam–sprayed casserole dish, add enough spaghetti sauce to barely cover bottom. Add stuffed shells. Cover with remaining sauce. Sprinkle with Parmesan cheese. Bake at 350° for 30 minutes or until bubbly.

Mom's Prize Winning Meat Loaf

1½ pounds ground round
1 cup tomato juice
¾ cup oats, uncooked
1 Egg Beater

¼ cup onion, chopped
1 teaspoon salt
¼ teaspoon pepper

Combine all ingredients; mix well. Press into a Pam–sprayed loaf pan. Bake at 350° for 1 hour. Let stand 5 minutes before cutting.

Pepper Steak

1½ pounds round steak, ½–inch thick
1 cup onions, sliced
1 cup beef broth
¼ cup celery, chopped
1 to 2 teaspoons salt or to taste
½ teaspoon sugar
½ teaspoon garlic powder
½ teaspoon ginger

2 green peppers, cut into strips
1 small can mushrooms
1 can stewed tomatoes
1 tablespoon soy sauce
2 tablespoons Lawry's stir fry sauce
2 tablespoons cornstarch
1 cup water

Brown steak in a Pam–sprayed Dutch oven. Add broth, onion, celery, salt, sugar, garlic and ginger; simmer, covered, for 35 to 40 minutes, or until tender. Add peppers, mushrooms and tomatoes; cook an additional 10 minutes. Mix soy sauce, Lawry's, cornstarch and water and stir until smooth. Slowly stir into meat mixture and cook, stirring constantly, until thickened. Serve over rice.

Quick Pepper Steak

1½ pounds boneless chuck
  steak
1 envelope Lipton onion soup
  mix
2 cups water

1 medium red pepper, chopped
1 medium green pepper,
  chopped
1½ tablespoons cornstarch
¼ cup cold water

Cut meat into thin strips about 2 inches long. In a large Pam–sprayed non–stick skillet brown meat, turning often; drain. Stir in soup mix and 2 cups water. Cover; simmer 30 minutes. Add peppers; cover and simmer 10 minutes or until meat is tender. Blend cornstarch with ¼ cup water. Stir into skillet. Cook, stirring constantly, until thick. May be served over rice.

Ship Wreck Casserole

1 can kidney beans
2 medium potatoes, diced
1 can carrots, drained
1 medium onion, diced

1 can tomato sauce
½ pound diet ground round
½ can tomato soup

Cook meat in a colander in microwave so that fat can cook out. Set aside. In a Pam–sprayed casserole dish layer vegetables in order given. Add tomato sauce then cooked meat. Top with tomato soup. Bake at 350°, covered, for 45 minutes. Check potatoes for doneness. Uncover and cook an additional 15 minutes.

Stuffed Peppers

2 pounds ground round
2 cups soft bread crumbs
¾ cup milk
2 Egg Beaters
½ cup onion, finely chopped
½ cup green pepper, finely
   chopped

6 to 8 bell peppers, halved
1 envelope Lipton's onion soup
   mix
2 tablespoons brown sugar
Pepper

Mix together all ingredients except the bell peppers that have been cut in half. Stuff meat mixture into green pepper halves. Place on a Pam–sprayed cookie sheet. Bake at 350° for 45 minutes to 1 hour, depending on size of peppers.

Spaghetti Casserole

1 envelope McCormick's
   spaghetti seasoning
1 (8–ounce) can tomato sauce
1½ cups water
2 teaspoons sugar
½ onion, chopped
½ bell pepper, chopped

½ pound healthy lean ground
   beef
Angel hair pasta
Fat–free Cheddar cheese,
   shredded
Parmesan fat–free cheese

Sauté onions and peppers in a non–stick Pam–sprayed skillet. Mix together seasoning packet, tomato sauce, water, sugar and sautéed vegetables. Cook ground beef in microwave and rinse. Add to sauce. Cook on medium until comes to a boil. Reduce heat and let slowly simmer for 2 to 3 hours. Cook pasta according to package directions. In a Pam–sprayed casserole dish, spoon a small amount of sauce into bottom of dish. Add a layer of pasta, sauce and then Cheddar cheese. Make another layer with pasta, sauce and top with Parmesan. Bake at 350° for 25 to 30 minutes or until bubbly.

Spicy Pot Roast

1 (3–pound) beef tenderloin
¼ cup wine vinegar
¼ cup ketchup
¼ cup Butter Buds Liquid
  (see page 50)
2 tablespoons soy sauce

2 tablespoons Worcestershire
  sauce
½ teaspoon garlic salt
1 teaspoon mustard
2 teaspoons minced onion

Brown roast on all sides. Combine all ingredients and pour over meat. Cover. Cook at 325° for 2 hours or until done and tender.

Veal Piccata

1 pound veal scaloppine
1 cup all–purpose flour
Salt and pepper to taste
3 to 4 cloves garlic, minced
½ pound fresh mushrooms,
  sliced
1 whole shallot, minced

3 tablespoons fresh lemon
  juice
¾ cup dry white wine
3 tablespoons dried parsley
3 to 4 teaspoons capers
3 teaspoons caper juice
½ lemon, sliced

Lightly dredge veal in flour. Sprinkle with salt and pepper. Brown veal in a non–stick Pam–sprayed skillet and set aside. Sauté mushrooms, garlic and shallot in a Pam–sprayed skillet. Add lemon juice, wine, parsley, capers and caper juice. Return veal to skillet. Simmer 15 to 20 minutes or until tender. Garnish with lemon slices.

Veal Scallopini

1½ pounds veal cutlets
¼ cup flour
1 teaspoon salt
Garlic powder to taste

2 whole cloves
1 can sliced mushrooms, liquid
  reserved
½ cup red wine

Cutlets should be thin. Rub cutlets with flour and sprinkle with salt, pepper and garlic. "Fry" in a Pam–sprayed non–stick skillet. Cook until browned. Stir in mushrooms with liquid and wine. Add cloves. Cover and simmer until liquid is reduced.

Veal Parmesan

6 to 8 veal cutlets
1 Egg Beater
Salt to taste
Pepper to taste
Bread Crumbs (seasoned)
   (see page 161)
¾ cup onion, chopped
½ cup green pepper, chopped
1 small jar sliced mushrooms
1 (6–ounce) can tomato paste

3 (8–ounce) cans tomato sauce
1 teaspoon garlic powder
3 bay leaves
1 tablespoon Italian seasoning
½ teaspoon oregano
2 tablespoons sugar
6 to 8 slices fat–free mozzarella
   cheese
Fat Free Parmesan cheese

Salt and pepper veal. Brush with Egg Beater. Roll in seasoned bread crumbs. Bake veal at 400° until done and browned. Sauté peppers and onions in a Pam–sprayed skillet. Add mushrooms, tomato paste, tomato sauce, garlic, bay leaves, Italian seasoning, oregano and sugar. Simmer for 30 minutes. In a Pam–sprayed casserole, spoon enough sauce to barely cover bottom. Add veal cutlets. Cover with mozzarella slices. Pour sauce over cutlets. Bake at 350° for 35 minutes. Sprinkle with Parmesan cheese before serving.

Lamb Shish Kabobs

Lean lamb, cut into 1–inch
   cubes
½ cup red wine
¼ cup water
1 teaspoon rosemary
1 clove garlic, minced

1 teaspoon Worcestershire
   sauce
2 tablespoons ketchup
1 teaspoon sugar
1 tablespoon white wine
   vinegar

Mix marinade ingredients and pour over lamb cubes. Marinate overnight. Place meat on skewers. Use remaining sauce for basting while grilling.

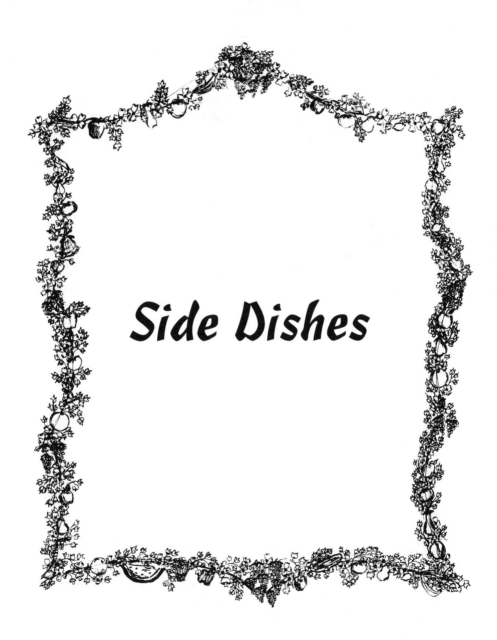

Side Dishes

Apple Pickles

4 to 6 apples
1 cup vinegar
1 cup water

2 cups sugar
Whole cloves

Put one clove in the bottom of each apple. Boil vinegar, water and sugar. Reduce heat and add apples. Cover; cook slowly until done. Remove cloves from apples before serving.

Baked Apples

6 McIntosh apples
½ teaspoon vanilla extract
1 cup sugar
4 tablespoons dark brown
  sugar

Ground cinnamon
1 lemon peel, cut in strips
3 tablespoons Fleischmann's
  Fat Free Squeezable Spread

Slice top and bottoms off of apples. Remove core and seeds. Lightly rub tops and bottoms with vanilla extract. Dip cut ends in bowl of sugar. Place apples, upright, in a Pam–sprayed shallow glass baking dish. Insert a piece of lemon peel into the center of each apple. Fill apple cavities with brown sugar. Sprinkle tops with cinnamon. Top each with ½ tablespoon Fleischmann's. Bake at 400° for about 20 minutes or until small cracks form on rims of apples.

"Fried" Apples

4 cups apples, peeled, cored
  and sliced
¼ cup + 1 tablespoon sugar
2 tablespoons Fleischmann's
  Fat Free Squeezable Spread

1 tablespoon Ultra Promise
  70% Less Fat
½ teaspoon cinnamon
½ cup water
¼ teaspoon salt

In a medium non–stick skillet place ingredients in same order listed. Cover and bring to a boil. Uncover and cook until liquid is reduced by half. Do not stir.

Artichoke Stuffing

1 large can artichoke hearts
⅓ cup fat–free Parmesan cheese
2 cups Italian Bread Crumbs
  (see page 161)
1 teaspoon minced garlic
1 teaspoon minced onion

¼ cup water
2 tablespoons Ultra Promise
  70% Less Fat
2 tablespoons Fleischmann's
  Fat Free Squeezable Spread
1 tablespoon fresh lemon juice

Drain artichokes, reserve liquid and slice thinly. Combine remaining ingredients, including liquid. Alternate layers of artichokes and bread crumb mixture, ending with bread crumbs. Bake at 325° for 20 minutes.

OR

Combine all ingredients and use in chicken, turkey or pork for stuffing.

Asparagus Casserole

1½ tablespoons Ultra Promise
  70% Less Fat
3 tablespoons Fleischmann's
  Fat Free Squeezable Spread
1 can Campbell's Healthy
  Request cream of mushroom
  soup

1 cup fat–free Cheddar cheese,
  grated
2 (#2) cans asparagus, drained
3 boiled egg whites, diced
Paprika

In a small saucepan, mix Promise, Fleischmann's, soup and cheese; simmer until cheese melts, stirring constantly. In a Pam–sprayed casserole dish, layer 1 can of asparagus, followed by half the egg whites and half of the soup mixture; repeat. Sprinkle with paprika. Bake at 350° for 25 minutes or until bubbly.

Baked Green Beans

2 (10–ounce) cans French style
  green beans
1 chicken bouillon cube
1 can Campbell's Healthy
  Request cream of chicken
  soup

½ teaspoon tarragon
½ cup evaporated skimmed
  milk
3 tablespoons Fleischmann's
  Fat Free Squeezable Spread
2 slices bread, cubed

Cook green beans with bouillon cube until well done. Drain. In a small mixing bowl mix together soup, tarragon, and milk. Fold into beans. Pour into a Pam–sprayed casserole dish and bake at 350° for 30 minutes. Mix together bread crumbs and Fleischmann's. Top green beans with bread mixture and bake an additional 12 minutes.

Black Beans on Rice

1 (12–ounce) package black
  beans
2 medium or 1 large green
  pepper, diced
1 cup onions, diced

½ teaspoon minced garlic
2 bay leaves
¼ cup distilled vinegar
Salt to taste
Rice, cooked

Wash beans. Add all ingredients, omitting rice, with enough water to cover. Cook covered until beans are tender, checking to make sure there is enough water. Remove 1 cup of beans and mash to make a gravy; return to pot. Serve over rice.

Creole Beans

1 slice Oscar Mayer bacon
2 (14½–ounce) cans French
  green beans
2 tablespoons dry onion soup
  mix

1 (16–ounce) can stewed
  tomatoes
1 teaspoon sugar
4 tablespoons Bacon Bits

Combine first 5 ingredients in a medium saucepan. Cook until beans are very tender. Top with Bacon Bits.

Country Green Beans

2 cans green beans
1 slice Oscar Mayer bacon
½ cup onion, coarsely chopped

1½ teaspoons sugar
½ teaspoon salt
¼ teaspoon pepper

In a saucepan, add bacon, onion, beans and remaining ingredients in that order. Heat to boil then reduce heat to slow simmer. Cook 1½ hours or until beans are done.

Easy Green Beans

3 (10–ounce) packages frozen French–style green beans, thawed
1 (8–ounce) can water chestnuts, drained and thinly sliced

3 tablespoons Ultra Promise 70% Less Fat
2 tablespoons Fleischmann's Fat Free Squeezable Spread
1 teaspoon rosemary

Combine all ingredients. Bake at 325°, covered, for 1 hour.

Fancy White Beans

½ pound dried white beans
2 quarts water
1 bay leaf
3 sprigs parsley
2 cloves garlic
½ tablespoon salt
1 medium onion, chopped

1¼ pounds ripe tomatoes, peeled, chopped and drained
¼ teaspoon dried sage
2 tablespoons tomato paste
Pinch of salt
Black pepper to taste

Soak beans overnight in enough water to cover. Next morning, drain. Add 2 quarts of water, bay leaf, parsley and garlic. Cover. Bake at 350° for 2 hours. Stir in salt and let bake 30 minutes longer. Sauté onions in a non–stick Pam–sprayed skillet. Add tomatoes to onions. Stir in sage and tomato paste and let simmer for 20 minutes. Season with salt and pepper. Drain beans; discard bay leaf, parsley and garlic. Combine with tomato mixture. Return to casserole and bake for 20 minutes. Serve hot.

Green Bean Casserole

2 cans French–style green
  beans
2 tablespoons Ultra Promise
  70% Less Fat, divided
1 tablespoon four
½ teaspoon salt
⅛ teaspoon pepper
2 teaspoons sugar
1 teaspoon onion flakes
1 tablespoon pimento
1 cup fat–free sour cream
½ cup fat–free Cheddar cheese,
  shredded
½ cup crushed corn flakes

Cook and drain green beans. Combine flour, 1 tablespoon Promise, salt, pepper and sugar; mix well. Add onion, pimento, sour cream and cheese. Add beans and mix well. In separate container add remaining Promise and corn flake crumbs. Place green bean mixture in a Pam–sprayed casserole dish and top with corn flake mixture. Bake at 350°, uncovered, for 25 minutes.

Green Bean Casserole Bake

2 cans green beans
1 tablespoon sugar
1 (5–ounce) can water chestnuts
1 (5–ounce) can mushrooms
1 medium onion, diced
1 can Campbell's Healthy
  Request cream of mushroom
  soup
1 can Campbell's Healthy
  Request cream of celery soup
1 cup fat–free Cheddar cheese,
  shredded
Salt and pepper to taste
Paprika

Cook beans with sugar and salt until tender; drain. Sauté onions in a non–stick Pam–sprayed skillet. In a medium saucepan heat soups and cheese just until cheese melts. In a Pam–sprayed casserole dish layer one half of the beans, chestnuts, mushrooms and onion. Cover with half the soup mixture. Repeat the layers. Sprinkle top with paprika. Bake at 350° for 30 minutes or until bubbly.

Green Beans with Mushrooms

2 garlic cloves, minced
1 medium red onion, cut in
   strips
¼ pound fresh mushrooms,
   trimmed and sliced

1 tablespoon Ultra Promise
   70% Less Fat
1 pound fresh green beans
1 teaspoon tarragon
Dash black pepper
Salt to taste

In a non–stick Pam–sprayed skillet, sauté garlic, onion and mushrooms; set aside. Steam beans until crisp tender. Combine beans and mushroom mixture; add tarragon, salt and pepper. Serve immediately.

Fordhook Lima Beans

2 (10–ounce) boxes frozen
   Fordhook limas
1 slice Oscar Mayer bacon

Salt and pepper to taste
1 teaspoon sugar

In a saucepan, place bacon on bottom, top with beans and add seasonings. Barely cover beans with water. Cover and simmer slowly for one hour or until tender. Discard bacon before serving.

Lima Beans with Mushrooms

2 (16–ounce) bags frozen lima
   beans
2½ tablespoons Ultra Promise
   70% Less Fat
1½ tablespoons Fleischmann's
   Fat Free Squeezable Spread

¼ pound fresh mushrooms,
   sliced
½ cup evaporated skimmed
   milk
Salt to taste
Pepper to taste

Cook lima beans in salted water until the beans are just tender. Sauté mushrooms in the Promise. Drain beans and add mushrooms, Fleischmann's, milk, salt and pepper. Heat through. Serve hot.

Refried Beans

1 pound dried pinto beans
2 beef bouillon cubes
1 onion, diced
1 teaspoon garlic powder
1 teaspoon salt
1 teaspoon pepper

½ cup fat–free Cheddar cheese,
  shredded
½ cup fat–free mozzarella
  cheese, shredded
1 teaspoon cumin

Cook beans in 5 cups cold water with bouillon cubes. When beans are almost done, add onion and spices. Continue to simmer beans until tender. Mash beans and onions with a potato masher or blend in blender. Continue cooking until beans are thickened. Mix cheese in the beans. Spread beans in a Pam–sprayed shallow pan. Bake at 350° for 15 minutes.

Snappy Green Beans

2 (#2) cans green beans
2 strips of Oscar Mayer bacon,
  divided
2 tablespoons pimento, diced
2 tablespoons red wine vinegar

2 teaspoons sugar, divided
1 tablespoon Worcestershire
  sauce
¼ teaspoon dry mustard
Salt and pepper to taste

Simmer beans with one slice bacon, 1 teaspoon sugar and salt for 45 minutes. Fry other slice of bacon until crisp then crumble. In a small saucepan add pimento, vinegar, sugar, Worcestershire and mustard. Boil, stirring constantly. Remove bacon from beans and discard. Drain beans. Add crumbled bacon and vinegar mixture. Mix well. Serve warm.

Spicy Baked Beans

2 cans vegetarian pork and
  beans, drained
¼ cup onion, finely diced
⅜ cup grape jelly

¼ cup hot enchilada sauce
1 slice Oscar Mayer bacon,
  halved

In a non–stick Pam–sprayed skillet sauté onions. Add jelly and enchilada sauce. Mix well. Add beans. Pour into Pam–sprayed casserole dish. Top with bacon. Bake at 350° for 1 hour.

If spicy taste is desired without the hot taste, use mild enchilada sauce.

White Beans

1 cup dried white beans
1 slice Oscar Mayer bacon
1 teaspoon salt

½ teaspoon pepper
Water

Wash and pick white beans. Place in medium saucepan with enough water to cover adequately. Add bacon. Cook, covered, over medium heat until boiling. Reduce heat and simmer for several hours until almost done. Add salt and pepper and continue cooking until completely tender. Discard bacon before serving.

Broccoli Casserole

2 (10–ounce) packages frozen
  chopped broccoli, cooked and
  drained
3 hard–boiled egg whites,
  sliced

1 cup fat–free sour cream
½ cup Weight Watcher's Fat
  Free Whipped Dressing
2 tablespoons tarragon vinegar
Paprika

Arrange broccoli in a Pam–sprayed 1½ quart shallow dish. Top with egg slices; set aside. In a small saucepan combine sour cream, whipped dressing and vinegar. Heat on lowest heat for 5 minutes, stirring constantly. Do not boil. Pour over broccoli. Bake, uncovered, at 350° for 10 minutes. Sprinkle with paprika.

Baked Broccoli Casserole

2 (10–ounce) packages frozen
　broccoli, cooked and drained
1 can Campbells's Healthy
　Request cream of celery soup
1 small jar pimento

1 can sliced water chestnuts,
　chopped
Bread Crumbs (see page 161)
1½ tablespoons Ultra Promise
　70% Less Fat

Mix together soup, pimento and chestnuts. Fold in broccoli. Place in a Pam–sprayed casserole dish. Top with bread crumbs that have been tossed with Promise. Bake at 350° for 30 minutes or until bubbly.

NOTE: You may add 2 cups cooked, chopped, skinless chicken breasts in mixture.

Company Broccoli

4 cups fresh broccoli, cut into
　flowerets
4 tablespoons onions, finely
　chopped
2 boiled egg whites, sliced
1 can water chestnuts, drained
　and chopped

1 can Campbell's Healthy
　Request cream of mushroom
　soup
1 cup fat–free Cheddar cheese,
　shredded
½ cup Weight Watcher's Fat
　Free Whipped Dressing
½ cup fat–free cracker crumbs

Cook broccoli according to package directions. Drain. Place broccoli in a Pam–sprayed casserole dish. Sprinkle with onion and layer with egg slices; top with water chestnuts. In a small saucepan, combine soup, cheese and whipped dressing. Cook over low heat until cheese is almost melted. Pour soup mixture over broccoli and sprinkle with cracker crumbs. Bake at 350° for 20 minutes or until bubbly.

Broccoli Rice Casserole

2 packages frozen, chopped
  broccoli, thawed
2 cans Campbell's Healthy
  Request cream of celery soup
2 cups Minute rice, uncooked
1 cup fat–free Cheddar cheese,
  shredded
¾ cup celery, chopped
¾ cup onion, chopped

1 cup evaporated skimmed
  milk
¼ cup Ultra Promise 70% Less
  Fat
⅛ cup Fleischmann's Fat Free
  Squeezable Spread
¼ cup Butter Buds Liquid
  (see page 50)

Combine all ingredients. Place in a Pam–sprayed casserole dish. Bake at 325°, covered, for 45 minutes. Uncover and bake an additional 15 minutes.

Creamy Broccoli Casserole

3 (10–ounce) packages frozen
  broccoli, cooked and drained
10 sliced Borden's Fat Free
  American cheese, diced
1 can Campbell's Healthy
  Request cream of mushroom
  soup

2 Egg Beaters
1 cup Weight Watcher's Fat
  Free Whipped Dressing
2 tablespoons onion, grated
Salt and pepper to taste
1 cup fat–free saltine cracker
  crumbs

Layer broccoli in a Pam–sprayed casserole dish. Layer with cheese. In a separate bowl, combine soup, Egg Beaters, whipped dressing, onion, salt and pepper. Spoon soup mixture over cheese. Bake at 350° for 20 minutes. Top with cracker crumbs and bake an additional 10 minutes or until bubbly.

Sweet and Sour Brussels Sprouts

3 cups fresh or 2 (9–ounce)
  packages frozen Brussels
  sprouts
2 slices Oscar Mayer bacon
¼ cup water
½ tablespoon Ultra Promise
  70% Less Fat

2 tablespoons vinegar
2 teaspoons sugar
½ teaspoon salt
¼ teaspoon garlic powder
⅛ teaspoon black pepper

Wash and trim Brussels sprouts. Cook 10 minutes or according to package directions. Drain. Fry bacon until crisp; drain well, crumble and set aside. In a small saucepan add water, Ultra Promise, vinegar, sugar, salt, garlic and black pepper. Cook to boiling. Add sprouts, stir and heat thoroughly. Serve topped with bacon.

Baked Celery

3 cups celery, cut into ½–inch
  pieces
1 teaspoon tarragon
½ cup evaporated skimmed
  milk

½ cup dry white wine
2 tablespoons Ultra Promise
  70% Less Fat

Combine ingredients in a Pam–sprayed casserole dish. Cover. Bake at 350° for 45 minutes.

Easy Cabbage

7 to 8 cups water, depending on
  size of cabbage
1 head cabbage, shredded
2 teaspoons beef bouillon

½ teaspoon black pepper
6 tablespoons sugar
1 tablespoon balsamic vinegar
Salt to taste

Bring water, sugar, salt, pepper, bouillon and vinegar to a boil. Add cabbage; cover and cook 8 to 10 minutes to crisp–tender. Leave top on cabbage until ready to serve.

Baked Cream Cabbage

1 medium head of cabbage
2 cups boiling salted water
3 tablespoons flour
1½ cups evaporated skimmed
  milk

Salt to taste
2 tablespoons Fleischmann's
  Fat Free Squeezable Spread
¼ cups bread crumbs

Finely shred cabbage. Cook in boiling water for 5 minutes. Remove cabbage and drain well. Place in Pam–sprayed casserole dish.

In small saucepan mix flour and 3 tablespoons milk; mix well until there are no lumps. Add remaining milk and Fleischmann's. Cook on low heat, stirring constantly until thick. Pour sauce over cabbage. Sprinkle with bread crumbs. Bake at 325° for 15 minutes.

Cabbage Pie

1 medium cabbage, thinly
  shredded

16 fat–free soda crackers,
  crumbled

WHITE SAUCE:
2½ tablespoons Ultra Promise
  70% Less Fat
4 tablespoons flour
½ teaspoon pepper

¼ teaspoon celery seed
1 teaspoon salt
2 cups skim milk
Paprika

Make a wine sauce by mixing Promise with flour, pepper, celery seed and salt. Stir until paste–like. Add milk whisking until smooth. Cook; whisking constantly until thick.

In a Pam–sprayed baking dish alternate layers of crumbled crackers and shredded cabbage, starting with cabbage and ending with crackers, making three layers of each. Pour white sauce over all. Bake at 350° for 45 minutes or until bubbly.

Carrots with Tarragon

12 to 14 carrots, sliced
  diagonally
2 teaspoons chicken flavor
  instant bouillon

2 tablespoons sugar
2 teaspoons Ultra Promise 70%
  Less Fat
½ teaspoon tarragon

In a medium saucepan, combine carrots, bouillon and sugar. Cook covered until crisp tender. Drain liquid; add Promise and tarragon; stir gently. Serve immediately.

Glazed Carrots

1 medium bunch carrots,
  peeled and sliced
2 tablespoons Ultra Promise
  70% Less Fat

⅓ cup brown sugar, firmly
  packed
½ teaspoon nutmeg
¼ cup fresh orange juice

Cook carrots until tender crisp. Mix together remaining ingredients. Add carrots. Cook, stirring until carrots are glazed. Serve immediately.

Jenny's Zesty Carrots

6 to 8 carrots, sliced
2 tablespoons onion, grated
1 tablespoon horseradish

½ cup Weight Watcher's Fat
  Free Whipped Dressing
¼ teaspoon salt
⅛ teaspoon pepper

Cook carrots; reserve ¼ cup water. Combine reserved water, onion, horseradish, whipped dressing, salt and pepper. Pour over carrots that have been placed in a Pam–sprayed casserole dish. Bake at 350° for about 20 minutes. Serve hot.

Cauliflower and Asparagus Casserole

1 (10–ounce) package frozen
  cauliflower
1 can asparagus
1 can Healthy Request cream of
  mushroom soup
1 cup fat–free Cheddar cheese,
  shredded

2 Egg Beaters
2 tablespoons pimento
1 teaspoon onion flakes
Salt to taste
Pepper to taste

Cook cauliflower according to directions on package and drain. Add together all ingredients. Pour into a Pam–sprayed casserole dish. Bake at 350° for 30 minutes or until bubbly.

Curried Cauliflower

2 (10–ounce) packages frozen
  cauliflower
½ teaspoon salt
1 can Campbell's Healthy
  Request cream of chicken
  soup

1 cup fat–free Cheddar cheese,
  shredded
⅓ cup Weight Watcher's Fat
  Free Whipped Dressing
1 teaspoon curry powder
⅛ cup bread crumbs
  (see page 161)

Cook cauliflower according to package directions; drain. Mix remaining ingredients and add to cauliflower. Sprinkle bread crumbs on top. Bake at 350° uncovered for 30 minutes or until bubbly.

Corn Casserole

1 can cream style corn
¼ cup onion, chopped
1 cup evaporated skimmed
   milk
¼ cup Egg Beater
4 tablespoons pimento,
   chopped

1 teaspoon Butter Buds Liquid
   (see page 50)
Salt and pepper to taste
1 cup fat-free crackers, crushed
I Can't Believe It's Not Butter
   spray

Sauté onions in a non-stick Pam-sprayed skillet. Mix together corn, onions, milk, Egg Beater, pimento, Butter Buds Liquid, salt and pepper. Pour into a Pam-sprayed casserole dish. Top with crackers. Lightly spray with butter spray. Bake at 350° for 45 minutes.

Succotash

2 cups whole kernel corn,
   frozen
2 cups baby lima beans, frozen
2 tablespoons sugar
1 teaspoon salt

¼ teaspoon pepper
½ cup evaporated skimmed
   milk
2 tablespoons Fleischmann's
   Fat Free Squeezable Spread

In a medium saucepan combine corn, beans, sugar and salt in enough water to cover. Cook until beans are tender. Drain. Add pepper, milk and Fleischmann's. Heat thoroughly. Serve hot.

Summer Corn Casserole

2 (10–ounce) cans whole kernel
  white corn, drained
1 (12–ounce) can French style
  whole green beans, drained
Salt and pepper to taste
1 can Campbell's Healthy
  Request cream of celery soup
1 (8–ounce) carton fat–free sour
  cream
1 onion, chopped
4 to 5 slices Borden's Fat Free
  American cheese slices, diced
15 reduced fat Ritz crackers,
  crushed
1 tablespoon Ultra Promise
  70% Less Fat

Layer beans and corn in a Pam–sprayed casserole dish; sprinkle with salt and pepper. Sauté onion in a Pam–sprayed skillet. Combine soup, sour cream, onion, and cheese. Pour soup mixture over corn. Bake at 300° for 35 minutes. Remove from oven and top with Ritz crackers and Promise. Return to oven and bake an additional 10 minutes.

Sweet Corn Pudding

3 Egg Beaters
3 tablespoons sugar
2 tablespoons Ultra Promise
  70% Less Fat, melted
2 tablespoons Fleischmann's
  Fat Free Squeezable Spread
½ cup evaporated skimmed
  milk
1 (16–ounce) bag frozen white
  whole kernel corn
¼ cup pimento, diced
2 tablespoons green pepper,
  chopped extra–fine
½ teaspoon salt or to taste
¼ teaspoon pepper

Combine Egg Beaters, sugar, Promise, Fleischmann's and milk, stirring well after each addition. Stir in remaining ingredients. Pour into Pam–sprayed casserole dish. Bake at 350° for 45 minutes or until set.

Cornbread Dressing

8 cups Cornbread, crumbled
  (see page 175 but omit sugar)
5 cups chicken broth
1 can Campbell's Healthy
  Request cream of chicken
  soup
2 teaspoons poultry seasoning

1 tablespoon sage (or to taste)
½ cup celery, chopped
⅔ cup onion, chopped
2 Egg Beaters
Salt and pepper to taste
Turkey Gravy (see page 83)

Mix dry ingredients. Add broth and soup. Mix well. Add Egg Beaters. Pour into a Pam–sprayed casserole dish. Bake at 350° for 1½ hours or until a knife inserted in middle comes out clean. Serve with Turkey Gravy.

Eggplant Parmesan

1 large eggplant
1 Egg Beater
1 cup dried Italian Bread
  Crumbs (see page 161)
½ cup fat–free Parmesan cheese
1 teaspoon oregano

1 teaspoon thyme
Salt
4 slices mozzarella fat–free
  cheese slices
3 (8–ounce) cans tomato sauce

Slice eggplant into ¼–inch thick slices. Boil until tender crisp. Brush each piece with Egg Beater then roll into bread crumbs. "Fry" in a non–stick Pam–sprayed skillet; turning once. Spray eggplant with Pam spray before turning. Cook until browned on both sides. Place a layer of eggplant in a Pam–sprayed 2 quart casserole dish; sprinkle with some of the thyme, salt, Parmesan and oregano. Place 2 slices of the cheese on top of eggplant. Cover with some of the tomato sauce. Repeat until all eggplant is used but leaving the mozzarella off of the top layer. Sprinkle Parmesan on top of last layer of sauce. Bake uncovered at 350° for 30 minutes or until bubbly.

Eggplant Soufflé

1 medium eggplant
2 tablespoons flour
1 cup fat–free Cheddar cheese,
  shredded
2 tablespoons Ultra Promise
  70% Less Fat

1 cup skim milk
3 Egg Beaters
3 egg whites
1 teaspoon salt
1 teaspoon pepper

Peel and slice eggplant. Boil until tender, about 10 minutes. Drain. Add salt and pepper. Mash until fine. Make a cream sauce by blending the Ultra Promise with flour and add milk; mix until smooth. Cook sauce, stirring constantly until thick; set aside and let slightly cool. Mix cream sauce with Egg Beater and eggplant. Beat egg whites until stiff. Fold eggplant mixture into egg whites. Add cheese. Spoon mixture into a Pam–sprayed 2 quart casserole. Bake at 350° for 40 to 45 minutes or until done.

Cheese Grits

1 cup grits
3 cups boiling water
Salt to taste
½ cup Butter Buds Liquid
  (see page 50)
1 tablespoon Ultra Promise
  70% Less Fat

6 slices fat–free American
  cheese, cubed
1 Egg Beater
2 ounces (or about 24 chips)
  Baked Lays Low Fat potato
  chips, crushed

Cook grits in salted boiling water for 5 minutes. Add Butter Buds Liquid, Promise, cheese and Egg Beater, stirring until cheese melts. Pour into a Pam–sprayed casserole dish. Top with crushed potato chips. Bake at 350° for 30 minutes.

VARIATIONS: Add ¼ to ½ teaspoon garlic to mixture for Garlic and Cheese Grits.

Spicy Cheese Grits

¾ cup white grits
3 cups water
¾ teaspoon salt
4 tablespoons Fleischmann's Fat Free Squeezable Spread
2 ounces Kroger's Classics sharp Cheddar cheese, shredded

½ cup fat–free Cheddar cheese, shredded
½ teaspoon Worcestershire sauce
2 Egg Beaters
1 (4–ounce) can chopped green chilies
Cayenne pepper to taste, optional

Cook grits in water and salt until done. Add Fleischmann's and cheeses. Stir until melted. Add Worcestershire. Fold in Egg Beaters and chilies. Pour into a Pam–sprayed 1½ quart baking dish. Sprinkle with cayenne. Bake at 350° for 45 minutes.

Turnip Greens

12 cups coarsely chopped turnip or mustard greens
1 cup water
1 beef bouillon cube

⅛ teaspoon crushed red pepper
1 slice Oscar Mayer bacon
¼ teaspoon salt
¼ teaspoon sugar

Combine all ingredients in a large Dutch oven. Cook slowly until tender. Water may need to be added, according to cooking temperature.

Gourmet Hominy Bake

1 (14–ounce) can hominy, drained and rinsed
1 (4–ounce) can green chilies
⅓ cup fat–free sour cream
¼ cup evaporated skimmed milk

½ cup fat–free mozzarella cheese, shredded
1½ tablespoons Ultra Promise 70% Less Fat
1 small jar pimento
1 teaspoon sugar

Mix all ingredients. Place in a Pam–sprayed casserole dish. Bake at 350° for 25 minutes.

Baked Macaroni and Cheese

2 cups small sea shell macaroni
Salt to taste
2 tablespoons Ultra Promise
  70% Less Fat
2 tablespoons Fleischmann's
  Fat Free Squeezable Spread

1½ cups fat–free Cheddar
  cheese, shredded
2 Egg Beaters
1½ cups evaporated skimmed
  milk

Cook macaroni and salt according to package directions and drain. Mix Ultra Promise, Fleischmann's, cheese, Egg Beaters and milk in a small saucepan. Cook just until cheese melts, stirring constantly. Add macaroni. Bake at 375° for 30 minutes.

Baked Onions

4 large onions
4 tablespoons brown sugar
4 teaspoons salt
2 teaspoons pepper

1 strip Oscar Mayer bacon
2 tablespoons Fleischmann's
  Fat Free Squeezable Spread

Peel onions and cut almost through in quarters. Place brown sugar, salt, pepper and Fleischmann's in onion. Top with ¼ strip bacon. Wrap in aluminum foil. Bake at 400° for 45 minutes or until tender crisp.

Fluffy Baked Onions

6 Egg Beaters
1 tablespoon flour
1 tablespoon cornstarch
1 cup skim milk

2 tablespoons Ultra Promise
  70% Less Fat
½ teaspoon salt
¼ teaspoon black pepper

Mix together flour, cornstarch, salt and pepper. Gradually add cold milk and mix until smooth. Beat egg whites until stiff. Mix Egg Beaters with milk mixture. Add egg whites and fold into milk mixture. Melt Promise in a heavy Pam–sprayed skillet. Pour in egg mixture. Bake at 350° for 20 minutes. Serve immediately.

Creamed Onions

2 pounds small white onions   ¾ cup water
½ teaspoon salt

Remove skins from onions. Place in a small saucepan; add salt and water. Simmer until tender crisp. Don't over cook. Drain. Prepare cream sauce.

CREAM SAUCE:
1 cup evaporated skimmed   1 tablespoon flour
  milk   1 bay leaf
1 tablespoon Ultra Promise   ½ teaspoon salt
  70% Less Fat

Mix together Promise and flour into a paste. Add milk whisking until mixture is smooth. Add bay leaf and salt. Cook on low; stirring constantly until thick. Cook for 5 minutes. Remove bay leaf. Add sauce to hot onions. Heat but do not boil. Serve immediately.

Onion Rings

1 jumbo sweet onion, sliced   1 envelope Shake–N–Bake
2 egg whites, beaten until   Country Mild for chicken
  foamy

Steam sliced onions over boiling water until softened, about 2 minutes. Plunge into cold water to stop cooking. Drain very well. Combine onions and egg whites. One at a time, roll onion ring into Shake–N–Bake. Shake off excess. Place on a Pam–sprayed baking sheet. Bake at 425° for 20 minutes, turning once. Eat immediately.

VARIATION: Substitute equal amounts of flour and Herb and Parmesan Cheese Potato Shakers in place of Shake–N–Bake Country Mild.

Onion Pie

2 cups onion, diced
5 Egg Beaters
¾ cup evaporated skimmed
  milk
¾ teaspoon salt
Dash pepper
1 tablespoon Ultra Promise
  70% Less Fat

1 tablespoon Fleischmann's Fat
  Free Squeezable Spread
¼ cup fat–free Cheddar cheese,
  shredded
¼ cup fat–free mozzarella
  cheese, shredded
1 Pie Crust (see page 327)

In a small Pam–sprayed skillet sauté onions. Mix Egg Beaters, milk, salt, pepper, Ultra Promise and Fleischmann's. Add onions and cheese. Pour into an uncooked pie crust. Bake at 350° for 30 minutes.

Black–eyed Peas

4 cups fresh or frozen black–
  eyed peas
Water
1 teaspoon salt

½ teaspoon pepper
1 teaspoon sugar
1 slice Oscar Mayer bacon

Combine all ingredients in medium saucepan. Cover with water. Cook until boiling; reduce heat and simmer until peas are tender.

Black–eyed Peas with Ham

2 cups dried black–eyed peas
3 chicken bouillon cubes
2 slices Oscar Mayer bacon
¼ cup onions
Salt to taste

Pepper to taste
1 tablespoon chopped red chili
  pepper
2 cups Healthy Choice ham,
  diced

In a large saucepan, combine black–eyed peas, bouillon, bacon, and enough water to generously cover peas. Bring to a boil and reduce heat to simmer for about 1½ hours or until peas are almost done. Add onions, salt, pepper, red pepper and ham. Cook an additional 30 minutes or until peas are completely done. Add more water if necessary during cooking.

Garden Style Oven Peas

2 (10–ounce) packages frozen
  green peas
1 (3–ounce) can sliced
  mushrooms, drained
¼ cup onions, chopped
¼ teaspoon salt

½ teaspoon basil
¼ cup Fleischmann's Fat Free
  Squeezable Spread
1 tablespoon water
⅛ teaspoon pepper

Sauté onions in a non–stick Pam–sprayed skillet. Mix all ingredients in a Pam–sprayed 1½ quart baking dish. Cover and bake at 350° for 1 hour, stirring occasionally.

Green Pea Casserole

1 cup onion, chopped
1 cup celery, chopped
1 cup green pepper, chopped
4 cups green peas, drained
1 cup sliced water chestnuts
  with liquid
1 small jar pimento

½ cup Butter Buds Liquid
  (see page 50)
1 can Campbell's Healthy
  Request cream of mushroom
  soup
Salt and pepper to taste
½ cup bread crumbs
  (see page 161)

Sauté onion, celery and pepper in a non–stick Pam–sprayed skillet. Mix together all ingredients excluding bread crumbs. Pour into a Pam–sprayed casserole dish and top with bread crumbs. Bake, uncovered, at 350° for 30 minutes or until bubbly.

Hoppin' John

2 cups turkey ham, diced into ¼–inch cubes	1 celery stalk, diced
1 bay leaf	½ teaspoon crushed red pepper
½ cup onions, chopped	Salt and pepper to taste
	2 cups black–eyed peas, dried
	2 cups rice, uncooked

Add bay leaf, onions, celery and seasonings. Discard any discolored or damaged peas and wash remaining peas. Add peas to pot. Cover with water. Simmer slowly until peas are tender. Cook rice separately. Add rice and ham to peas. Heat thoroughly. Serve hot.

Candied Yams

2 (23–ounce) cans yams, sliced	¼ teaspoon nutmeg
½ cup brown sugar	2 tablespoons Ultra Promise 70% Less Fat
1 tablespoon + 2 teaspoons flour	1 tablespoon Fleischmann's Fat Free Squeezable Spread
¼ teaspoon salt	1 cup orange juice
¼ teaspoon cinnamon	

In a small mixing bowl mix together sugar, flour, salt, cinnamon and nutmeg; set aside. Place half of the sliced yams in a Pam–sprayed casserole dish. Sprinkle with half of the sugar mixture. Dot with Fleischmann's. Add the remaining yams and sprinkle with remaining sugar mixture. Add orange juice. Dot with all the Ultra Promise. Bake at 350° for 45 minutes.

Butterscotch Yams

6 medium–sized yams, cooked,
  peeled and halved
1 cup packed light brown sugar
½ cup dark corn syrup

¼ cup evaporated skimmed
  milk
3 tablespoons Fleischmann's
  Fat Free Squeezable Spread
½ teaspoon salt

In a heavy pan mix sugar, corn syrup, milk, Fleischmann's and salt; bring to a boil, stirring constantly. Cook for 5 minutes on medium heat. Place yams in a Pam–sprayed casserole dish. Pour sauce over potatoes. Bake at 350° for 20 to 25 minutes.

Fried Potato Patties

2 cups leftover Mashed
  Potatoes (see page 265)
¼ cup onion, finely diced
⅛ cup green pepper, finely
  diced

⅛ cup Egg Beater
1 tablespoon parsley flakes
½ cup self–rising flour
⅛ cup self–rising cornmeal

Mix all ingredients together. Pam–spray a moderately hot (not extremely hot) non–stick skillet. Drop batter by spoonsful in skillet, mashing down to form a patty. Cook until browned. Spray each patty with Pam before turning. Turn over and cook other side. Continue until all mixture is used.

Fancy New Potatoes

16 new potatoes
2 tablespoons Ultra Promise
  70% Less Fat

4 tablespoons Fleischmann's
  Fat Free Squeezable Spread
¼ cup parsley, minced

Wash potatoes. Boil in salted water until tender. Drain. Toss with Promise, Fleischmann's and parsley.

Glazed Sweet Potato & Apple Casserole

4 medium–sized sweet potatoes
2 large apples
½ teaspoon salt
2 teaspoons lemon juice
2 tablespoons Ultra Promise
   70% Less Fat

1 tablespoon Fleischmann's Fat
   Free Squeezable Spread
⅓ cup molasses
¼ cup brown sugar
2 tablespoons white sugar
Butter salt to taste
Apple pie spice to taste

Boil sweet potatoes until tender but still firm; allow to cool. Peel and slice. Place in a Pam–sprayed baking dish. Core and slice apples and sprinkle with lemon juice. Sauté apples in Ultra Promise until slightly soft. Arrange apples with sweet potatoes. Add Fleischmann's to molasses. Pour over apples and potatoes. Sprinkle with salts, sugars and apple pie spice. Bake at 325° for 30 minutes.

Helen's Potatoes au Gratin

5 medium potatoes, diced
2 tablespoons Ultra Promise
   70% Less Fat
2 tablespoons flour
1 teaspoon salt
½ teaspoon pepper

1 cup evaporated skimmed
   milk
½ cup fat–free Cheddar cheese,
   shredded
½ cup fat–free cracker crumbs

Arrange potatoes in a Pam–sprayed casserole dish. Combine Promise and flour to make a paste. Whisk in milk, salt and pepper. Heat, whisking until warm. Add cheese; stir until cheese melts. Pour sauce over potatoes. Top with cracker crumbs. Bake at 350° for 30 minutes.

Mashed Potatoes

4 cups potatoes, peeled, diced,
   cooked and drained
½ cup fat–free chicken broth

Salt to taste
White pepper to taste

Mash potatoes with an electric mixer. Add broth, salt and pepper. Continue beating until smooth. Serve hot.

Onion–Roasted Potatoes

2 pounds potatoes, cut into
   bite–size pieces

1 envelope onion soup mix
Pam butter spray

After potatoes are diced, spray with Pam butter spray until well coated. Add soup mix and toss until potatoes are coated. Empty potatoes into a Pam–sprayed shallow dish. Bake at 425°, stirring occasionally, 30 minutes or until potatoes are tender and golden brown.

Potato–Mushroom Bake

4 cups potatoes, pared and
   sliced
1 cup onion, peeled and sliced
2 cups fresh mushrooms, sliced

¾ teaspoon salt
¼ teaspoon black pepper
1 teaspoon dried tarragon
   leaves
¼ cup water

In a Pam–sprayed shallow baking dish, layer potatoes, onion and mushrooms. Sprinkle with salt, pepper and tarragon. Pour in water. Cover with foil. Bake at 350° for 30 minutes. Remove foil; continue baking until potatoes are fork tender. Serve immediately.

Potatoes Romanoff

6 medium potatoes, peeled and
   diced
2 cups fat–free sour cream
1½ cups fat–free Cheddar
   cheese, shredded

1½ teaspoons salt
¼ teaspoon pepper
1 bunch green onions, chopped
Paprika

Sauté onions in a non–stick Pam–sprayed skillet. Boil potatoes until fork tender. Mash; stir in sour cream, cheese, salt, pepper and onions. Pour into Pam–sprayed casserole dish. Top with paprika. Cover and refrigerate overnight. Bake uncovered at 350° for 30 to 40 minutes. Let set for 15 minutes before serving.

Scalloped Potatoes

½ cup Campbell's Healthy
   Request cream of mushroom
   soup
½ cup skim milk
1 tablespoon Ultra Promise
   70% Less Fat
4 cups potatoes, peeled and
   thinly sliced

¼ cup green pepper, chopped
¼ cup onions, chopped
½ teaspoon salt
⅛ teaspoon pepper
I Can't Believe It's Not Butter
   spray

Mix soup, milk and Promise; heat but do not boil. Alternate two layers of potatoes, peppers and onions in a Pam–sprayed casserole dish. Season both layers with salt, pepper and butter spray. Pour heated soup mixture over all. Cover. Bake at 350° for 1½ hours. Uncover and cook an additional 30 minutes.

Skillet Potatoes

1 tablespoon Ultra Promise
   70% Less Fat
1 cup onions, chopped
½ cup Weight Watchers Fat
   Free Whipped Dressing
¼ cup cider vinegar
1 tablespoon sugar

1¾ teaspoons salt
¼ teaspoon pepper
4 medium potatoes, peeled,
   sliced and cooked
1 slice Oscar Mayer bacon,
   cooked crisp, drained and
   crumbled

In a non–stick Pam–sprayed skillet, sauté onions. Add Promise, whipped dressing, vinegar, sugar, salt and pepper. Stir in potatoes; cook, stirring constantly, 2 minutes or until hot. DO NOT BOIL. Top with cooked bacon pieces.

Stewed Potatoes

5 cups potatoes, diced
1 small onion, largely diced
½ slice Oscar Mayer bacon
½ cup evaporated skimmed
 milk
1 tablespoon Ultra Promise
 70% Less Fat

1 tablespoon Fleischmann's Fat
 Free Squeezable Spread
Salt to taste
Pepper to taste
1½ tablespoons cornstarch
1½ tablespoons water

In a medium saucepan add potatoes, onion, bacon, salt and pepper. Scarcely cover with water. Cover. Simmer until almost done. Add Promise, Fleischmann's and milk. Continue to simmer until potatoes are completely done. Mix together cornstarch and water. Add to simmering potatoes and cook, stirring until thick.

Stuffed Sweet Potatoes

6 medium sweet potatoes
⅛ cup Ultra Promise 70% Less
 Fat
⅛ cup Butter Buds Liquid
 (see page 50)
⅓ cup sugar

1 Egg Beater
½ teaspoon cinnamon
½ teaspoon allspice
¼ teaspoon salt
½ cup miniature marshmallows

Bake potatoes at 400° for 1 hour. Cool; cut potato in half. Scoop out potato, leaving shell. Mash and stir in all ingredients omitting marshmallows. Spoon back into shells.

Bake at 350° for 15 minutes. Remove from oven. Top with marshmallows and return to oven for an additional 10 minutes or until marshmallows are golden brown.

Sweet Potato Croquettes

2 cups fresh sweet potatoes,
  cooked, mashed (DO NOT
  USE CANNED)
1¼ tablespoons brown sugar

1 tablespoon Ultra Promise
  70% Less Fat
1 teaspoon vanilla extract
1 Egg Beater
1 cup graham cracker crumbs

Mix first 4 ingredients well. Pat into patties. Brush with Egg Beater. Roll into graham cracker crumbs. Place on a Pam–sprayed cookie sheet. Bake at 350° for 15 minutes. Turn and bake an additional 15 minutes or until golden.

Sweet Potato Bake

2 tablespoons Ultra Promise
  70% Less Fat
2 tablespoons Fleischmann's
  Fat Free Squeezable Spread
1½ cups raw sweet potato,
  grated

3 Egg Beaters
½ cup brown sugar
⅓ cup white sugar
¾ cup evaporated skimmed
  milk
Pinch of salt

Combine all ingredients. Pour into a Pam–sprayed loaf pan. Bake at 350° for 1½ hours, or until set.

Sweet Potato Custard

1 cup sweet potatoes, peeled,
  cooked and mashed
2 small bananas, mashed
1 cup skim milk
2 tablespoons brown sugar

1 tablespoon sugar
¼ teaspoon cinnamon
½ teaspoon salt
2 Egg Beaters
3 tablespoons raisins

Combine potatoes and bananas. Add milk and blend. Add remaining ingredients. Pour into Pam–sprayed 1–quart casserole dish. Bake at 300° for 45 minutes until custard is firm and golden. Serve with lamb or pork.

Twice–Cooked Potatoes

6 medium potatoes
3 tablespoons Ultra Promise
  70% Less Fat
3 tablespoons Fleischmann's
  Fat Free Squeezable Spread
2 cups fat–free Cheddar cheese,
  shredded

2 cups fat–free sour cream
1½ teaspoons salt
⅛ teaspoon pepper
1 cup onion
Paprika

Boil potatoes in skins. Refrigerate overnight. Peel potatoes and grate them. Mix together all ingredients. Place in a Pam–sprayed 2–quart casserole. Bake at 350° for 45 minutes.

Potato and White Cheese Casserole

8 medium sized potatoes
1 cup evaporated skimmed
  milk
2 Egg Beaters
1½ cups fat–free mozzarella
  cheese, shredded

2 tablespoons Fleischmann's
  Fat Free Squeezable Spread
Salt to taste
Pepper to taste

Peel and boil potatoes until tender. Drain and mash. Add milk; mix well. Add Egg Beaters and cheese. Season with salt, pepper and Fleischmann's. Place in a Pam–sprayed casserole dish. Bake at 450° for 15 minutes or until golden.

Rosemary Potatoes

6 baking potatoes
2 tablespoons rosemary
1 envelope dry onion soup mix

2 egg whites, slightly beaten
Butter salt

Wash potatoes and slice into ½–inch rounds. Combine rosemary and soup mix. Dip potatoes in egg whites then toss in dry seasoning. Place in single layer in a Pam–sprayed baking dish. Sprinkle with butter salt. Cover and bake at 350° for 1 hour.

Whipped Potatoes

4 cups potatoes, peeled and
  diced
½ cup evaporated skimmed
  milk

1 tablespoon Ultra Promise
  70% Less Fat
2 tablespoons Fleischmann's
  Fat Free Squeezable Spread
Salt and pepper to taste

Cook potatoes with salt until done; drain. Add milk, Promise and Fleischmann's. With an electric mixer, beat until smooth. Add salt and pepper.

Baked Rice with Cheese

2 cups rice, cooked
4 Egg Beaters
1½ cups skim milk
1½ cups fat–free Cheddar
  cheese, shredded

2 tablespoons Ultra Promise
  70% Less Fat
4 tablespoons Fleischmann's
  Fat Free Squeezable Spread
½ teaspoon mustard

Melt cheese, Promise, Fleischmann's and milk in a double boiler. Mix remaining ingredients. Add this to cheese mixture. Place in Pam–sprayed casserole dish. Bake at 325° for 1 hour.

Curried Rice

1 cup raw rice
2 small apples, peeled, cored
  and chopped
1 tablespoon Ultra Promise
  70% Less Fat
½ cup onion, finely chopped

¼ teaspoon garlic powder
½ tablespoon curry powder
½ bay leaf
1½ cups chicken broth
Salt to taste

Sauté onion in a non–stick Pam–sprayed skillet; add apple and curry powder. Stir to mix. Add rice, bay leaf, broth and salt. Stir; bring to a boil. Cover and simmer for 20 minutes or until done. Remove bay leaf and fluff with fork.

Herbed Rice

1 cup onion
1 tablespoon Ultra Promise
  70% Less Fat
1 cup raw rice
3 cups fat–free chicken broth
¾ teaspoon basil

¾ teaspoon marjoram
½ teaspoon sage
¼ teaspoon thyme
¼ teaspoon curry powder
½ teaspoon salt

In a Pam–sprayed skillet, sauté onion. Add remaining ingredients. Bring to a boil, cover and cook over a low heat for 30 minutes or until broth is absorbed and rice is cooked.

Luncheon Rice

2 cups rice
1 package frozen broccoli,
  chopped
2 Egg Beaters
1 cup onion, chopped
3 tablespoons Ultra Promise
  70% Less Fat

1 tablespoon Fleischmann's Fat
  Free Squeezable Spread
½ teaspoon garlic, minced
1 cup skim milk
¾ cup fat–free Cheddar cheese,
  shredded
Salt to taste
Pepper to taste

Cook rice according to package omitting margarine. Sauté onions in a Pam–sprayed skillet. Cook and drain broccoli. Combine all ingredients. Bake in a Pam–sprayed casserole dish at 350° for 45 to 50 minutes.

Seasoned Rice

1 cup white rice
2½ cups fat–free chicken broth
1½ teaspoons Lawry's seasoned
   salt or to taste
2 tablespoons Ultra Promise
   70% Less Fat

2 tablespoons Fleischmann's
   Fat Free Squeezable Spread
½ cup green pepper, diced
½ cup green onions, including
   tops, chopped
3 tablespoons pimento, diced

Cook rice in broth with seasoned salt. In a Pam–sprayed skillet, sauté onions and peppers. Add Ultra Promise, Fleischmann's, onions, peppers and pimentos to rice.

Spanish Rice

1 medium onion, chopped
1 teaspoon garlic powder
1 cup long grain rice
¾ cup Rotel
2 beef bouillon cubes

2½ cups water
¾ teaspoon cumin
1 tablespoon sugar
2 tablespoons tomato paste
Salt to taste

Sauté onion in a non–stick Pam–sprayed skillet. Combine all ingredients. Bring to a boil, cover, reduce heat and simmer over very low heat until liquid is reduced and rice is tender, approximately 20 minutes.

Skillet Spinach

1 (10–ounce) package frozen
   spinach
Seasoning salt to taste

2 Egg Beaters
¼ cup fat–free Parmesan cheese

Cook spinach in a non–stick Pam–sprayed hot skillet. Cook 3 minutes, stirring constantly. Add Egg Beaters and salt, stirring constantly. Sprinkle with cheese.

Spinach Casserole

2 (10–ounce) boxes frozen
chopped spinach
1 cup fat–free Swiss cheese,
grated or sliced

¼ cup evaporated skimmed
milk
1 teaspoon rosemary
Salt and pepper to taste

Cook spinach, drain well and place in a shallow Pam–sprayed baking dish. Cover with cheese and milk. Sprinkle with rosemary, salt and pepper. Place under broiler until cheese melts and thoroughly heated.

Debbie's Squash Casserole

8 yellow squash, washed and
sliced
1 onion, chopped
1 green pepper
2 tablespoons Fleischmann's
Fat Free Squeezable Spread

4 ounces Velveeta light
2 Egg Beaters
50 fat–free saltines, crushed
Salt and pepper to taste

Boil squash, onion and green pepper until tender; drain well. Add remaining ingredients. Bake at 350° for 40 to 45 minutes or until firm.

Easy Broiled Zucchini

3 small, thin zucchini
1 teaspoon salt
¼ teaspoon pepper

½ cup fat–free Parmesan cheese
Fleischmann's Fat Free
Squeezable Spread

Slice zucchini into ¼–inch rounds. Arrange closely in a single layer Pam–sprayed cookie sheet. Dot each piece with Fleischmann's. Sprinkle with salt and pepper. Generously sprinkle with cheese. Broil about 7 minutes or until lightly browned but tender crisp. Serve immediately.

Butternut Bake

1 large butternut squash (about
   2½ pounds)
2 tablespoons Ultra Promise
   70% Less Fat
2 tablespoons Fleischmann's
   Fat Free Squeezable Spread
1 tablespoon brown sugar
¼ teaspoon salt
Dash of pepper

Cinnamon
¼ cup sugar
1½ quarts Jonathan apples,
   peeled, cored and diced
1 cup corn flake crumbs
2 tablespoons Fleischmann's
   Fat Free Squeezable Spread
1 cup brown sugar
Butter salt

Cut squash in half lengthwise; remove seeds. Bake, face down in shallow pan of water at 350° for 30 minutes. Scrape out pulp and mash with a mixer until smooth. Add Promise, Fleischmann's, brown sugar, salt and pepper; set aside.

In a non–stick Pam–sprayed skillet add apples and sugar. Cover and simmer until just barely tender. Spoon apples in a Pam–sprayed casserole dish. Cover with squash. In a small bowl add corn flake crumbs, Fleischmann's and brown sugar. Top casserole with mixture. Sprinkle with butter salt. Bake at 350° for 15 to 20 minutes or until thoroughly heated.

Baked Squash with Blueberries

4 acorn squash
1 (12–ounce) container
   blueberries, fresh or frozen
1 apple, peeled and finely
   diced, divided
8 tablespoons brown sugar

8 teaspoons Ultra Promise 70%
   Less Fat
4 tablespoons Fleischmann's
   Fat Free Squeezable Spread
Salt
Allspice

Cut squash in half so edges are scalloped; remove seeds. Sprinkle squash with salt. Generously sprinkle each with allspice. Spoon berries into each squash half. Add apple. Sprinkle 1 tablespoon brown sugar over berries. Top with 1 teaspoon Ultra Promise and ½ tablespoon Fleischmann's. Put in a pan; add ¾ cup water. Cover. Bake at 375° for 45 minutes. Uncover and cook additional hour or until liquid in squash is reduced and squash is done.

Harvest Baked Squash

3 acorn squash
1 cup water
1 (13½–ounce) can crushed
  pineapple, drained
1½ cups apple, cored and diced
1 cup celery, diced
½ cup brown sugar

½ teaspoon cinnamon
¼ teaspoon salt
6 teaspoons Ultra Promise 70%
  Less Fat
3 tablespoons Fleischmann's
  Fat Free Squeezable Spread
Butter salt

Cut squash in half so edges are scalloped; remove seeds. Bake in water, cut side down at 350° for 45 minutes. Remove water from pan. In a small bowl add pineapple, apple, celery, brown sugar, cinnamon and salt; mix well. Sprinkle squash with salt. Spoon pineapple mixture into squash centers. To each squash half add 1 teaspoon Ultra Promise and ½ tablespoon Fleischmann's. Bake at 350° for an additional 45 minutes.

Jane's Squash Casserole

2 (10–ounce) packages frozen
  squash
1 cup onion, chopped
1 (8–ounce) carton fat–free sour
  cream
1 can Campbell's Healthy
  Request cream of chicken
  soup, undiluted

1 (8–ounce) can water
  chestnuts, sliced and drained
1 package chicken stuffing mix
¼ cup Butter Buds Liquid
  (see page 50)
2 tablespoons Ultra Promise
  70% Less Fat

Cook squash as according to package; drain. Sauté onions in a Pam–sprayed skillet. Combine squash, onions, sour cream, soup and chestnuts. Mix stuffing with Butter Buds Liquid and Promise. Add ¾ of stuffing mixture to squash mixture. Spoon into a Pam–sprayed casserole dish. Top with remaining stuffing mix. Bake at 350° for 20 minutes or until thoroughly heated.

Sherried Zucchini

4 small zucchini, sliced
¼ teaspoon dill weed
¼ teaspoon celery seed
1 teaspoon salt

1 teaspoon garlic powder
¼ cup dry sherry
Pepper to taste

Sprinkle dill, celery seed and salt over zucchini. Let stand for 10 minutes. In a non–stick Pam–sprayed skillet add zucchini, garlic, sherry and pepper. Cover and simmer only until zucchini softens.

Simple Baked Butternut

2 medium butternut squash
8 tablespoons sugar
Cinnamon

4 tablespoons Fleischmann's
    Fat Free Squeezable Spread
Butter salt

Cut squash in half lengthwise; remove seeds. Bake, cut side down, in shallow pan of water at 350° for 30 minutes. Remove squash from pan and turn cut side up. Sprinkle with butter salt. Top each with 1 tablespoon Fleischmann's; generously sprinkle with cinnamon. Top each with 2 tablespoons sugar. Bake at 350° for 50 minutes.

Skillet Squash

4 cups sliced squash
2 tablespoons diced onion
1 tablespoon sugar
Scant of salt

Pepper to taste
Water to barely cover
1 tablespoon Fleischmann's Fat
    Free Squeezable Spread

Add first 6 ingredients in a non–stick skillet and let cook, covered, until squash is tender. DO NOT STIR. Take top off; add Fleischmann's and cook until liquid is almost gone. DO NOT STIR.

Squash au Gratin

2 cups squash, sliced
¼ cup onion, chopped
2 tablespoons Ultra Promise
   70% Less Fat
2 tablespoons Fleischmann's
   Fat Free Squeezable Spread

¾ cup fat–free Cheddar cheese,
   shredded
2 Egg Beaters
Bread Crumbs (see page 161)
Salt to taste
Pepper to taste
2 teaspoons sugar

Boil squash until done, then mash. In a Pam–sprayed skillet sauté onions; add squash, Promise, Fleischmann's, cheese and Egg Beaters. Add 1 tablespoon bread crumbs. Pour into Pam–sprayed casserole dish. Sprinkle with bread crumbs. Bake at 325° for 1 hour.

Summer Squash

6 yellow summer squash,
   sliced
1 cup Weight Watcher's Fat
   Free Whipped Dressing
1 cup fat–free Parmesan cheese

1 teaspoon sage
½ teaspoon white pepper
1 cup onion, chopped
2 Egg Beaters

Mix together whipped dressing, cheese, sage, pepper, onion and Egg Beaters. Fold in squash. Place in a Pam–sprayed casserole dish. Bake at 350°, covered, for 1 hour.

Baked Tomatoes with Horseradish Mayonnaise

8 firm medium to small
   tomatoes
1 cup grated onion
½ cup brown sugar

Salt to taste
Paprika
Horseradish Mayonnaise
   (see page 60)

Slice tops off tomatoes. Scrape out seeds and watery material. Place 1 tablespoon onion on top and in cavity of each tomato. Place 1 tablespoon brown sugar on top of each. Top each tomato with desired amount of Horseradish Mayonnaise. Sprinkle with paprika. Bake at 450° for 8 minutes.

Corn Stuffed Tomatoes

8 to 10 medium tomatoes
3 slices Oscar Mayer bacon
1 (12–ounce) can whole kernel
    corn
¼ cup green onion, sliced
½ cup celery, chopped

½ cup Bread Crumbs
    (see page 161)
1 cup fat–free Cheddar cheese,
    shredded
1 teaspoon salt
1 teaspoon sugar

Wash tomatoes, cut off tops, hollow out and save pulp. Leave shell. Place in a shallow baking dish and set aside. Cook bacon crisp; crumble and set aside. Combine all ingredients including tomato pulp. Stuff into tomato shells. Bake at 350° for 20 minutes. Serve immediately.

Oven–Baked Fried Tomatoes

6 to 8 green tomatoes
1 Egg Beater
Bread Crumbs (see page 161)

Lawry's seasoned salt
Pepper

Wash tomatoes and slice into ½–inch slices. Dip tomato slices in Egg Beater and roll in crumbs seasoned with seasoned salt and pepper.

For crispy tomatoes, broil for 2½ minutes; turn over and broil another 2 minutes.

OR

Bake at 450° for 8 minutes.

Country Turnips

6 cups turnips, peeled and diced
1¼ cups water
1 strip Oscar Mayer bacon
½ teaspoon salt
3 tablespoons sugar
¼ teaspoon pepper

Mix all ingredients in a saucepan. Cover. Bring to a slow simmer. Cook until turnips are tender. Discard bacon before serving.

Fresh Vegetable Stir-Fry

2 tomatoes, chopped
½ cup carrots, grated
¾ cup broccoli flowerets
5 mushrooms, sliced
½ cup onion, chopped
1 large squash, sliced
1 large zucchini, sliced
¼ teaspoon rosemary
Teriyaki sauce
½ cup white wine
Rice, cooked
Fat-free Parmesan cheese

Prepare vegetables. Spray non-stick skillet or wok with Pam. Shake teriyaki sauce 5 times into skillet; add wine. Add vegetables and cook on high until heated thoroughly, no more than 5 minutes. Stir frequently. To serve, layer rice and vegetables and top with Parmesan cheese.

Vegetable Bake

1 can Veg-All, drained
½ cup celery, chopped
½ cup onion, chopped
½ cup water chestnuts, sliced
  and drained
1 cup Weight Watcher's Fat
  Free Whipped Dressing
1 cup Healthy Request cream
  of mushroom soup
1 cup fat-free Cheddar cheese,
  shredded
24 Low Fat or Fat Free
  Snackwell's crackers, crushed
I Can't Believe It's Not Butter
  spray

Mix first 7 ingredients well. Place in a Pam-sprayed casserole dish. Bake at 300° for 30 minutes. Remove from oven; add crackers and spray with butter spray. Return to oven and continue baking for an additional 15 minutes.

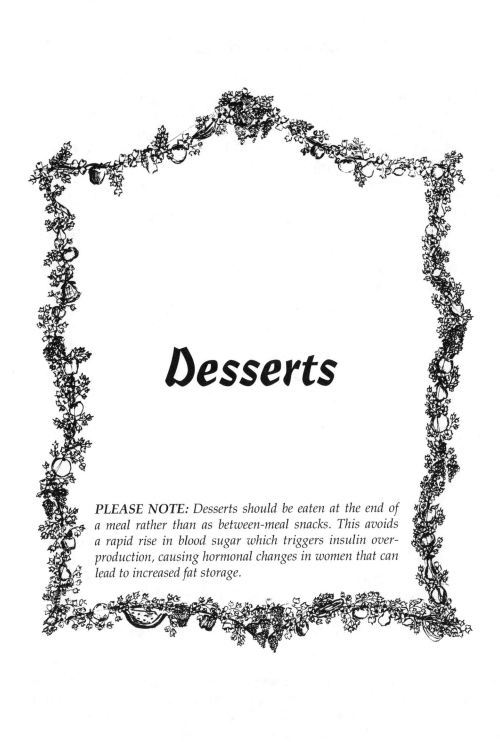

Desserts

PLEASE NOTE: *Desserts should be eaten at the end of a meal rather than as between-meal snacks. This avoids a rapid rise in blood sugar which triggers insulin over-production, causing hormonal changes in women that can lead to increased fat storage.*

Banana Meringue Pie

¾ cup sugar
3 tablespoons cornstarch
2 cups skim milk
3 Egg Beaters
Scant salt
1 tablespoon Ultra Promise
  70% Less Fat

1 teaspoon vanilla extract
2 bananas, sliced
1 (9–inch) Pie Shell, cooked
  (see page 327)
1 Meringue (see page 327)

Line the bottom of cooked pie shell with sliced bananas. Set aside. In a medium saucepan, combine sugar and cornstarch. Add milk, Egg Beaters and salt. Cook over medium heat, stirring constantly, until very thick. Remove from heat; add Promise and vanilla. Pour into pie shell. Top with Meringue.

Blueberry Heaven Pie

1 (21–ounce) can blueberry pie
  filling
3 cups Dream Whip, prepared
  (see page 329), or Cool Whip
  Free

1½ cups marshmallow creme
¼ teaspoon lemon peel, grated
Pinch of salt
1 Pie Shell, baked (see page 327)

Pour pie filling into prepared crust. Combine remaining ingredients and spoon over pie. Chill.

Butterscotch Meringue Pie

1 cup brown sugar
3 tablespoons cornstarch
2 cups skim milk
3 Egg Beaters
Scant salt
2 tablespoons Ultra Promise
  70% Less Fat

¼ cup Fleischmann's Fat Free
  Squeezable Spread
1 teaspoon vanilla extract
1 (9–inch) Pie Shell, cooked
  (see page 327)
Meringue (see page 327)

In a medium saucepan, add sugar and cornstarch. Add milk, Egg Beaters and salt. Cook over medium heat, stirring constantly until very thick. Remove from heat. Add Promise, Fleischmann's and vanilla. Pour into pie shell. Top with Meringue.

Chocolate A La Menthe Miniatures

1 (3.4–ounce) package chocolate
   instant pudding
1 cup skim milk

1½ tablespoons creme de
   menthe
30 Athen's mini fillo shells
Cool Whip Lite

Mix together milk and pudding, beating thoroughly. Add creme de menthe; mix well. Refrigerate until set. Fill fillo shells. Dot with Cool Whip Lite.

Chocolate Chess Pie

3 tablespoons Ultra Promise
   70% Less Fat
1 tablespoon Fleischmann's Fat
   Free Squeezable Spread
1½ cups sugar
3 tablespoons cocoa
5 ounces evaporated skimmed
   milk

2 Egg Beaters
1 teaspoon vanilla extract
Pinch of salt
1 teaspoon cornstarch
1 (9–inch) unbaked Pie Shell
   (see page 327)

Mix dry ingredients. Add remaining ingredients. Pour into pie shell and bake at 325° for 46 minutes. Serve with dollop of Cool Whip Lite.

Chocolate Delight Miniatures

1 (3.4–ounce) package chocolate
   instant pudding
1 cup skim milk

2 tablespoons Triple Sec
30 Athen's mini fillo shells
Cool Whip Free

Mix together milk and pudding, beating thoroughly. Add Triple Sec; mix well. Refrigerate until set. Fill fillo shells. Dot with Cool Whip Free.

Chocolate Meringue Pie

1 cup sugar
3½ tablespoons cocoa
6 tablespoons flour
Scant of salt
2 cups skim milk
2 Egg Beaters

2 tablespoons Ultra Promise
  70% Less Fat
1 teaspoon vanilla extract
1 (9–inch) Pie Shell, cooked
  (see page 327)
Meringue (see page 327)

Combine dry ingredients. Add milk and Egg Beaters. Bring to a boil over medium heat, stirring constantly. Boil for 2 minutes. Remove from heat. Add Promise and vanilla. Pour into pie shell. Top with meringue.

Cherries Jubilee Pie

2 egg whites
⅛ teaspoon cream of tartar
Dash of salt

½ cup sugar
½ teaspoon vanilla extract

Add salt and cream of tartar to unbeaten egg whites. Beat until they form soft peaks. Add sugar, 2 tablespoons at a time, beating well after each addition. Continue beating until stiff peaks form. Fold in vanilla. Spread mixture on bottom and sides of a Pam–sprayed and well floured pie plate. Bake at 325° for 30 minutes or until shell feels firm and dry. Cool.

SAUCE:
1 (1 pound 14 ounce) can pitted
  black sweet cherries
1 tablespoon cornstarch
Dash of salt

¼ cup sugar
1 tablespoon Ultra Promise
  70% Less Fat
2 teaspoons lemon juice

Drain cherries and save juice. Mix together in saucepan the cornstarch, salt and sugar. Add 1 cup cherry juice and mix well. Cook and stir over medium heat until mixture comes to a boil, then simmer 3 minutes. Remove from heat. Add Ultra Promise and lemon juice. Cool. Add cherries.

To serve: Fill shell with fat–free strawberry ice cream. Cut into pie shaped pieces and serve with sauce.

Chess Pie

3 Egg Beaters
1½ cups sugar
2 tablespoons Ultra Promise
   70% Less Fat
¼ cup + ⅛ cup Fleischmann's
   Fat Free Squeezable Spread

1 teaspoon vanilla extract
1 tablespoon vinegar
1 tablespoon cornmeal
½ tablespoon cornstarch
1 Pie Shell (see page 327)

Mix together all ingredients, mixing well. Pour into unbaked pie shell. Bake at 350° for 45 minutes or until set.

Country Pear Pie

1 cup sugar, divided
¼ teaspoon nutmeg
½ teaspoon cinnamon
2 tablespoons cornstarch
6 cups sliced pears
½ cup syrup from pears

2 tablespoons Ultra Promise
   70% Less Fat
2 tablespoons sugar
Pastry for 2 crust pie
   (see page 326)

Cook sliced pears and ¼ cup sugar in enough water to barely cover. Cook until tender. Mix ¾ cup sugar, nutmeg, cinnamon, cornstarch and Promise together. Make a paste with sugar mixture and syrup. Toss lightly with cooked pears. Spoon into prepared pie crust. Cover with top crust and cut a slit. Sprinkle with 2 tablespoons sugar. Bake at 425° for 30 to 35 minutes or until done.

Individual Caramel Tarts

2 packages Athen's mini fillo
   dough shells (15 each)

1 can fat–free Eagle Brand milk
Lite Cool Whip

Place unopened can of Eagle Brand milk in boiling water. Boil for 2 hours. Cool in refrigerator. Open and fill each shell ¾ full. Top each with a very small amount of Cool Whip.

Coconut Meringue Pie

⅓ cup + 2 tablespoons sugar
¼ cup cornstarch
¼ teaspoon salt
2¾ cups skim milk
2 drops yellow food coloring
1 tablespoon Ultra Promise
   70% Less Fat

1 tablespoon Fleischmann's Fat
   Free Squeezable Spread
1 teaspoon vanilla extract
¼ teaspoon butter extract
¼ teaspoon coconut extract
1 (9–inch) Pie Crust
   (see page 327)
Meringue (see page 327)

Add sugar and cornstarch. Gradually stir in milk. Bring to a boil over medium heat, stirring constantly. Boil 1 minute. Stir in remaining ingredients. Pour into the pie shell. Top with meringue.

Custard Pie

1 cup Egg Beaters
¾ cup sugar
¼ teaspoon salt
½ teaspoon vanilla extract
⅛ teaspoon almond extract

2½ cups skim milk, scalded
1 teaspoon cornstarch
Nutmeg
1 (9–inch) Pie Shell, unbaked
   (see page 327)

Blend Egg Beaters, sugar, salt, and extracts. Gradually stir in milk and cornstarch. Pour into pie shell. Sprinkle with nutmeg. Bake at 400° for 25 minutes. Turn oven off and let pie remain inside until oven is cool.

Fudge Pie

1 cup sugar
2 Egg Beaters
2 teaspoons cornstarch
3 tablespoons cocoa
½ cup evaporated skimmed milk

3 tablespoons Fleischmann's
   Fat Free Squeezable Spread
Pinch of salt
1 Pie Shell, unbaked
   (see page 327)

Mix above ingredients and pour into pie shell. Bake at 350° for 30 minutes or until knife inserted in middle comes out clean.

Key Lime Pie

½ cup Key lime juice
Fat–free Eagle Brand milk
Dash of salt
1 drop of green food coloring

3 cups Dream Whip, prepared
(see page 329), or Cool Whip
Free
1 Graham Cracker Crust
(see page 326)

Beat lime juice, milk, salt and food coloring until thoroughly combined. Fold in Dream Whip or Cool Whip Free and blend well. Pour into prepared crust and chill thoroughly.

Lemon Cheesecake

4 Egg Beaters
1 can fat–free Eagle Brand milk

Juice of 4 large lemons

Mix together well. Pour into a Pam–sprayed pie pan. Bake at 350° for 20 to 23 minutes.

Lemon Cheesecake Pie

1 (8–ounce) package fat–free
cream cheese, softened
1 can fat–free Eagle Brand milk
⅓ cup fresh lemon juice
1 teaspoon vanilla extract

1 tablespoon fat–free sour
cream
1 Graham Cracker Crust
(see page 326)

Beat cheese until fluffy; add Eagle Brand milk; blend thoroughly. Add lemon juice, vanilla and sour cream. Beat until creamy. Pour into crust. Let set at least 2 hours before cutting.

Lemon Cream Cheese Pie

1 can fat–free Eagle Brand milk
½ cup lemon juice, freshly
   squeezed
2 (8–ounce) packages fat–free
   cream cheese
1 Egg Beater
1 teaspoon vanilla extract

2 teaspoons cornstarch
2 tablespoons sugar
1 tablespoon fresh lemon peel
1 Graham Cracker Crust
   (see page 326)
1 can pie filling of choice, for
   topping

Whip cream cheese until smooth. In separate bowl mix together remaining ingredients. Gradually blend this mixture into cream cheese, beating thoroughly. Pour into pie crust and refrigerate until set. Top with pie filling.

Lemon Custard Pie

4 Egg Beaters
¾ cup sugar
2 tablespoons flour
1½ cups non–fat buttermilk
2 tablespoons Ultra Promise
   70% Less Fat
2 tablespoons Fleischmann's
   Fat Free Squeezable Spread

Grated peel of 1 lemon
3 tablespoons fresh lemon
   juice
1 teaspoon vanilla extract
1 (9–inch) Pie Shell
   (see page 327)
Cinnamon

Beat Egg Beaters and sugar together in large mixer bowl until light. Beat in flour, buttermilk, Promise, Fleischmann's, lemon peel, lemon juice and vanilla. Pour into pie shell. Sprinkle lightly with cinnamon. Bake at 375° for 30 minutes or until knife blade inserted near center comes out clean. Refrigerate before serving.

Lemon Ice Box Pie

1 cup fat–free Eagle Brand milk
1 can lemonade, undiluted
2 envelopes Dream Whip,
   prepared (see page 329), or
   Cool Whip Free

1 Graham Cracker Crust
(see page 326)

Mix together Eagle Brand milk and lemonade. Fold in Dream Whip or Cool Whip Free. Pour into a graham cracker crust. Cover and refrigerate until set.

Lemon Pie

4 Egg Beaters
2 cups sugar
½ cup lemon juice
¼ cup flour

1 teaspoon baking powder
Fillo mini shells or 1 Meringue
   Shell (see page 327)

Mix together Egg Beaters, sugar, lemon juice and flour. Stir in baking powder. Pour into a Pam–sprayed pie plate. Bake at 350° for 18 to 20 minutes. When cooled spoon into fillo shells or 1 baked meringue shell.

Lemon Pie Filling

4½ tablespoons fresh lemon
   juice
1 tablespoon lemon peel,
   grated
2 tablespoons Ultra Promise
   70% Less Fat

2 tablespoons Fleischmann's
   Fat Free Squeezable Spread
¾ cup sugar
3 tablespoons flour
1½ cups boiling water
3 to 4 drops yellow food
   coloring

In a medium saucepan make a paste with Promise, Fleischmann's and flour. Add boiling water and whisk briskly to remove all lumps. Add lemon juice, peel, sugar and food coloring. Stir over low heat until thick. Set aside and let cool or fill pie shell or pastries. Chill.

Lime Cream Cheese Pie

1 can fat–free Eagle Brand milk
½ cup lime juice, freshly
  squeezed
2 (8–ounce) packages fat–free
  cream cheese
¼ cup Egg Beaters
1 teaspoon vanilla extract

2 tablespoons sugar
1 tablespoon fresh lime peel,
  grated
2 teaspoons cornstarch
1 Graham Cracker Crust
  (see page 326)

Whip cream cheese until smooth. In separate bowl mix together remaining ingredients. Gradually blend this mixture into cream cheese, beating thoroughly. Pour into pie crust and refrigerate until set.

Lime Parfait Pie

1 (3–ounce) package lime
  gelatin
1 cup boiling water
¼ cup frozen lemonade
  concentrate, thawed

1 pint fat–free vanilla ice cream
1 Graham Cracker Crust
  (see page 326)

Dissolve gelatin in boiling water. Add lemonade. Add ice cream, stirring until melted and smooth. Chill mixture until it begins to thicken, about 20 minutes. Pour into pie shells. Freeze at least 3 hours before serving.

Mincemeat Pie

1 (9–ounce) Crosse & Blackwell
  mincemeat with rum &
  brandy
2 cups apples, peeled, cored
  and thinly sliced

2 tablespoons lemon juice
¼ cup sugar
1 Fat Free Pie Crust for bottom
  (see page 327)
1 Top Pie Crust (see page 327)

Combine mincemeat, apples, lemon juice and sugar. Fill uncooked fat free pie crust with filling. Adjust top crust and crimp edges. Sprinkle lightly with sugar. Bake at 400° for 25 minutes or until golden. May be served with Brandy Sauce (see page 72).

Luncheon Strawberry Pie

1 (3–ounce) package strawberry
   gelatin
1 cup boiling water
¼ cup fat–free sour cream
1 teaspoon lemon juice

1 (10–ounce) package frozen,
   sliced strawberries with
   sugar, thawed
Meringue Pie Shells, made for
   individual (see page 327)
Cool Whip Lite

Dissolve gelatin in water. Chill until syrupy. Beat at high speed of electric mixer until frothy. Blend in sour cream, lemon juice and strawberries. Refrigerate until partially set. Spoon into meringue shells. Top with dollop of Cool Whip.

Mrs. Minor's Pineapple Pie

1 cup sugar
3 tablespoons cornstarch
2 cups skim milk
2 Egg Beaters
1 cup crushed pineapple,
   drained

½ teaspoon vanilla extract
2 tablespoons Ultra Promise
   70% Less Fat
1 Pie Shell, baked (see page 327)
1 Meringue (see page 327)

In the top of a double boiler, mix together sugar, cornstarch, milk and Egg Beaters. Cook over medium heat. Add pineapple and cook until thickened. When thick, remove from heat and add vanilla and Promise. Pour into baked shell. Top with meringue. Bake at 350° for 10 minutes or until golden.

Pineapple Meringue Pie

1 cup sugar
3 tablespoons cornstarch
2 cups skim milk
3 Egg Beaters
Scant salt
1 tablespoon Ultra Promise
 70% Less Fat

1 tablespoon vanilla extract
1 small can crushed pineapple,
 drained
1 (9–inch) Pie Shell, baked
 (see page 327)
1 Meringue (see page 327)

In a medium saucepan, combine sugar and cornstarch. Add milk, Egg Beaters and salt. Cook over medium heat, stirring constantly until very thick. Remove from heat; add Promise, vanilla and pineapple. Pour into pie shell. Top with meringue.

Sour Cream Cheese Pie

1 can fat–free Eagle Brand milk
1 teaspoon cornstarch
⅓ cup lemon juice, freshly
 squeezed
¼ cup Egg Beaters
2 tablespoons sugar

¾ cup fat–free sour cream
1½ cups Dream Whip, prepared
 (see page 329), or Cool Whip
 Free
1 Graham Cracker Crust
 (see page 326)

Mix milk, cornstarch, lemon juice, Egg Beaters and sugar together thoroughly. Fold in sour cream and Dream Whip or Cool Whip Free. Pour filling in crust. Sparingly sprinkle crumbs on top; chill thoroughly.

Sour Cream Lime Pie

1 can fat–free Eagle Brand milk
⅓ cup lime juice, freshly
 squeezed
¼ cup Egg Beaters
2 tablespoons sugar
¾ cup fat–free sour cream

1½ cups Dream Whip, prepared
 (see page 329), or Cool Whip
 Free
1 Graham Cracker Crust
 (see page 326)

Mix milk, lime juice, Egg Beaters and sugar together thoroughly. Fold in sour cream and Dream Whip or Cool Whip Free. Pour filling in crust. Sparingly sprinkle crumbs on top; chill thoroughly.

Strawberry Banana Pie

1 (8–ounce) package fat–free
   cream cheese
¾ cup confectioners sugar
½ teaspoon vanilla extract
2 medium bananas, sliced
1 pint strawberries, thinly sliced

1 (8–ounce) package Dream
   Whip, prepared (see page
   329), or Cool Whip Free
1 Graham Cracker Crust
   (see page 326)

With a mixer, beat cream cheese, sugar and vanilla. Divide evenly
and set aside. On the graham cracker crust make a layer of bananas
using one whole banana and half of the strawberries; layer half of
cream cheese mixture; layer of 1 whole banana, remainder of cream
cheese mixture and ending with a layer of remaining strawberries,
placed on top in a decorative manner. Let chill thoroughly before
serving.

Strawberry Pie

1 cup sugar
1 cup water
4 tablespoons flour
½ teaspoon salt
Juice of 1 lemon
½ teaspoon red food coloring

2 pints strawberries, washed
   and capped
1 Pie Shell (see page 327)
   or 1 Graham Cracker Crust
   (see page 326)

Place prepared strawberries in desired pie shell. Mix first 4 ingredients and cook until thick. Remove from heat. Add lemon and coloring, stirring well. Let cool slightly. Pour over strawberries. Refrigerate.

Sweet Potato Pie

3 medium sweet potatoes,
  cooked and mashed
¼ cup evaporated skimmed
  milk
¼ cup skim milk
3 Egg Beaters
1 cup sugar
1 tablespoon flour

2 tablespoons Ultra Promise
  70% Less Fat
6 tablespoons Fleischmann's
  Fat Free Squeezable Spread
1 teaspoon vanilla extract
1 Pie Shell put in a deep dish
  pan, uncooked (see page 326)

Mix together first 9 ingredients. Pour into prepared pie shell. Bake at
350° for 40 minutes or until done.

Vanilla Surprise Miniatures

1 (3.4–ounce) package vanilla
  instant pudding
1 cup skim milk

2 tablespoons Grand Marnier
30 Athen's mini fillo shells
Cool Whip Lite

Mix together milk and pudding; beat thoroughly. Add Grand
Marnier. Refrigerate until set. Fill fillo shells. Top with a dot of Cool
Whip Lite.

Apple Bread Pudding

⅔ cup flour
¼ teaspoon salt
2 Egg Beaters
1¼ cups sugar

2 cups apple, peeled and
  chopped
1 teaspoon vanilla

Beat Egg Beater and sugar until smooth. Add flour and salt. Fold in
apples and vanilla. Spoon into 4 Pam–sprayed ramekin cups. Bake at
325° for 25 minutes.

Baked Alaska

3 (½–inch) thick slices Entenmann's Fat Free Golden loaf	6 egg whites ½ cup sugar
Fat–free chocolate, strawberry and vanilla ice cream	Scant of salt ½ teaspoon vanilla extract Hershey's chocolate syrup

Cut golden loaf with 2½–inch biscuit cutter. You should get 2 cuts per slice of loaf. Place in aluminum foil muffin cup. Scoop the fat–free ice creams so that all 3 flavors are equally present per scoop. Place these on top of cake rounds. Freeze.

Beat egg whites and salt until stiff; add sugar 1 tablespoon at a time, beating well after each addition. Add vanilla. Quickly cover each one with meringue and return to freezer for at least 3 hours.

Preheat oven to 450°. Remove Alaska from freezer and bake 2 to 3 minutes or until slightly brown. Top each with warm chocolate syrup. Serve immediately.

Blackberry Cobbler

¾ cup self–rising flour	½ teaspoon vanilla extract
1 cup sugar, divided	¼ cup skim milk
¼ cup Butter Buds Liquid (see page 50)	1 (16–ounce) can water packed blackberries

Pour berries and juice in the bottom of casserole dish. Sprinkle ¼ cup sugar on berries. Meanwhile, combine remaining sugar with the remaining ingredients; mix well. Pour batter on top of berries. Do not stir. Bake at 350° for 40 minutes or until done.

Bread Pudding

1 loaf French bread	1 teaspoon cinnamon
4 cups skim milk	1 cup raisins
3 Egg Beaters	3 tablespoons Fleischmann's
2 cups sugar	Fat Free Squeezable Spread
2 tablespoons vanilla extract	Bourbon Sauce (see page 71)

Cut bread into bite–size pieces. Place in large bowl and let sit uncovered, overnight. Cover with milk and soak 1 hour. Mix well. Add Egg Beaters and sugar; mix well. Add vanilla, cinnamon, raisins and Fleischmann's. Pour into a Pam–sprayed 9 x 13–inch pan. Bake at 375° for 50 minutes. Serve with Bourbon Sauce.

Cherry Delight

½ angel food cake, cubed	8 ounces fat–free sour cream
1 (3–ounce) box instant vanilla	1 can cherry pie filling
pudding	Dream Whip, prepared (see
1 cup skim milk	page 329), or Cool Whip Free

Place cake cubes in the bottom of a 9 x 13–inch pan. In a separate bowl, mix together pudding with the 1 cup milk; fold in sour cream. Spread mixture on top of cake. Spoon pie filling over pudding. Top with prepared Dream Whip or Cool Whip Free. Keep refrigerated.

Chocolate Peppermint Mousse

1 (3–ounce) package instant	1 cup Dream Whip, prepared
chocolate pudding	(see page 329), or Cool Whip
1½ cups skim milk	Free
15 hard peppermint candies	Cool Whip Lite

Beat pudding and milk until thick. Process candies in blender until powder. Pour into pudding mix. Fold in Dream Whip or Cool Whip Free. Refrigerate. When ready to serve, spoon into dessert dishes; serve with a dollop of Cool Whip Lite.

Chocolate Mousse

1 (8–ounce) package fat–free
   cream cheese
1¼ cups Domino chocolate
   flavored confectioners sugar

2 cups Dream Whip, prepared
   (see page 329), or Cool Whip
   Free

With a mixer, beat cream cheese until smooth. Add sugar; beat well.
Fold in Dream Whip or Cool Whip Free.

Company Bread Pudding

9 slices whole wheat bread,
   including crusts, broken into
   pieces
5 cups evaporated skimmed
   milk
4 Egg Beaters
½ cup sugar
½ cup brown sugar

2 teaspoons cinnamon
¼ teaspoon allspice
¼ teaspoon nutmeg
½ teaspoon salt
1 cup crushed pineapple,
   drained
2 bananas, sliced
½ cup raisins

Combine first 9 ingredients in a large bowl and let stand 30 minutes.
Stir in pineapple, banana and raisins. Pour into Pam–sprayed casserole dish. Bake at 375° for 40 minutes.

Easy Brownies

3 cups Pioneer low–fat biscuit
   mix
2 cups Domino chocolate
   flavored confectioners sugar

2 Egg Beaters
¼ cup skim milk
¼ cup Ultra Promise 70% Less
   Fat, melted

Stir together biscuit mix and sugar. Mix together Egg Beaters, milk
and Promise. Pour into a 9 x 9–inch Pam–sprayed pan. Bake at 350°
for 15 to 18 minutes or until done.

Four Layer Surprise

¾ cup Fleischmann's Fat Free
  Squeezable Spread
3 tablespoons Ultra Promise
  70% Less Fat
1 cup flour
4 ounces fat–free cream cheese
¾ cup confectioners sugar,
  divided

4 cups Dream Whip, prepared
  (see page 329), or Cool Whip
  Free, divided
1 (3–ounce) package instant
  chocolate pudding, or
  pudding of choice
1½ cups skim milk

Mix together Promise and flour; add Fleischmann's. Mix well. Pat into 9 x 9–inch Pam–sprayed dish. Bake at 375° for 10 minutes. Set aside. Mix together cream cheese and ½ cup sugar. Fold in 2 cups Dream Whip, prepared, or Cool Whip Free. Pour this mixture on top of cooked crust. Let set. Mix together instant pudding, ¼ cup sugar and skim milk. Pour this mixture on top of cream cheese mixture. Let set. Add remaining Dream Whip, prepared, or Cool Whip Free, on top. Keep refrigerated.

Grand Marnier Soufflé

Pam butter spray
Sugar
6 Egg Beaters
6 egg whites
½ cup sugar

¼ cup orange juice
3 tablespoons Grand Marnier
1 tablespoon fresh lemon juice
Grand Marnier Sauce
  (see page 75)

Pam–butter spray 6 individual 4–inch soufflé dishes. Sprinkle each dish with 1 teaspoon sugar, shaking out excess sugar. Combine Egg Beaters, sugar, orange juice and liqueur and whisk just until blended. Beat egg whites with 1 tablespoon sugar until soft peaks form. Add lemon juice and thoroughly blend. Fold egg mixture into whites. Spoon into soufflé dishes. Bake at 450° until puffed and browned, about 11 minutes. Remove dishes from oven; cut hole in top of soufflé and top with Grand Marnier Sauce.

Gimmie's Rice Custard

6 Egg Beaters
3 cups skim milk
1 cup sugar
1 teaspoon vanilla extract

½ teaspoon salt
1 teaspoon cinnamon (optional)
1 cup light raisins
1½ cups cooked rice

Pour Egg Beaters into a 2–quart casserole; beat slightly. Add milk, sugar, vanilla, salt and cinnamon. Blend well. Stir in rice and raisins. Set casserole in pan of water. Bake, uncovered, at 350° for 1 hour and 15 minutes, stirring once after 30 minutes.

Jan's No–Cook Banana Pudding

1 (6–ounce) package instant
vanilla pudding
2½ cups skim milk
1 (14–ounce) can fat–free Eagle
Brand milk

2 packages Dream Whip,
prepared (see page 329), or
Cool Whip Free
Reduced fat vanilla wafers
8 bananas

Mix together pudding and skim milk; add Eagle Brand milk. Fold in Dream Whip or Cool Whip Free. Layer wafers, bananas and pudding. Repeat until all is used.

Jane's Apple Crisp

8 tart apples, cored and sliced
⅔ cup sugar
½ teaspoon salt
¼ teaspoon cinnamon
2 tablespoons lemon juice
¼ cup Fleischmann's Fat Free
Squeezable Spread

1 cup flour
½ cup brown sugar
⅛ cup Ultra Promise 70% Less
Fat
⅛ cup Fleischmann's Fat Free
Squeezable Spread

Place prepared apples in a Pam–sprayed deep dish. Mix the next 4 ingredients and sprinkle over apples. Dot with Fleischmann's. Blend last 4 ingredients and cut to crumb–like consistency. Sprinkle evenly on top. Bake at 400° for 30 minutes.

Key Lime Mousse

1 tablespoon unflavored
  gelatin
1 cup sugar
¼ teaspoon salt
2 Egg Beaters
½ cup Key lime juice
¼ cup water

1 teaspoon lime peel, grated
Green food coloring
1 cup Dream Whip, prepared
  (see page 329), or Cool Whip
  Free
2 egg whites

Mix first 3 ingredients and set aside. In a saucepan, combine Egg Beaters, lime juice and water. Add gelatin mixture and cook until mixture boils, stirring constantly. When boiling, remove from heat. Add peel and just enough food coloring to make a pale green; chill, stirring occasionally. Do not let mixture get too cold and start to jell. Fold ½ cup Dream Whip or Cool Whip Free into gelatin mixture. Beat egg whites until stiff. Fold in egg whites. Pour into glasses and refrigerate. Top with dollop of remaining Dream Whip or Cool Whip Free.

Lemon Sponge Custard

1½ tablespoons Ultra Promise
  70% Less Fat
1 cup sugar
3 tablespoons flour
3 Egg Beaters

3 egg whites
1 tablespoon grated lemon rind
¼ cup lemon juice
⅛ teaspoon butter flavor extract
1½ cups skim milk

Cream Promise and sugar; add flour and Egg Beaters; stir. Add lemon rind, lemon juice, extract and milk. Beat egg whites until stiff; fold into batter mix. Pour into custard cups that have been sprayed with Pam. Bake at 425° for 10 minutes; reduce heat to 325° and bake 18 minutes more or until set.

Lemon Mousse

1 (8–ounce) package fat–free
   cream cheese
1¼ cups Domino lemon
   flavored confectioners sugar

2 cups Dream Whip, prepared
   (see page 329), or Cool Whip
   Free

With a mixer, beat cream cheese until smooth. Add sugar; beat well.
Fold in Dream Whip.

Marge's Cranberry Dessert

1 cup Quaker oats
½ cup all–purpose flour
1 cup brown sugar
3 tablespoons Ultra Promise
   70% Less Fat

5 tablespoons Fleischmann's
   Fat Free Squeezable Spread
1 can whole cranberry sauce

Cut Promise into oats, flour, and sugar. Add Fleischmann's. Sprinkle
½ mixture on bottom of a Pam–sprayed casserole dish. Spoon cranberry sauce over mixture. Top with remaining oat mixture. Bake at
350° for 40 minutes.

Peach Cobbler

1 cup self–rising flour
1 cup sugar
½ Butter Buds Liquid
   (see page 50)

1 teaspoon vanilla extract
½ cup skim milk
1 (29–ounce) can sliced peaches

In a small mixing bowl combine first 5 ingredients; mix well. Pour
mixture into a 9 x 13–inch Pam–sprayed casserole dish. Pour peaches
with juice on top. Do not stir. Bake at 350° for 47 to 50 minutes or
until done.

Raspberry Trifle

1 (13.6–ounce) Entenmann's Fat
  Free Golden loaf
2 cups red raspberry preserves
2½ to 5 ounces Royale Deluze
  Chambord liqueur
2 tablespoons sugar

½ cup sugar
1 tablespoon cornstarch
2 Egg Beaters
2¼ cups skim milk
½ teaspoon vanilla extract
Scant of salt

Slice pound cake and spread with preserves; cut in cubes. Place in a covered air tight container and pour raspberry liqueur over cubes. Cover and set overnight. Combine sugar and cornstarch. Whisk in Egg Beaters until you have a paste. Gradually whisk in milk to prevent lumps. Cook on medium heat, whisking continually until thick. Remove from heat and whisk in vanilla and salt. Cover and refrigerate.

Next day, place layer of cake in trifle bowl. Pour custard over layer. Make 2 layers. May be topped with fresh raspberries and Dream Whip, prepared, or Cool Whip Free.

Shortcake

2 cups all–purpose flour
¼ teaspoon salt
4 teaspoons baking powder
4 tablespoons sugar, divided in
  half

2 tablespoons Ultra Promise
  70% Less Fat
2 tablespoons Fleischmann's
  Fat Free Squeezable Spread
1 Egg Beater
½ cup skim milk

Mix all dry ingredients. Cut Ultra Promise into flour mixture. Add remaining ingredients. Lightly knead. Roll out to 1–inch thickness. Cut with biscuit cutter. Sprinkle top with remaining sugar. Place on Pam–sprayed cookie sheet. Bake at 425° for 8 to 10 minutes. Slice open and serve with fresh fruit and Dream Whip, prepared, or Cool Whip Free.

Strawberry Mousse I

1 (10–ounce) package frozen
  strawberries
¼ cup confectioners sugar
1 tablespoon lemon juice

¼ cup Cointreau liqueur
1 cup Dream Whip, prepared
  (see page 329), or Cool Whip
  Free

Crush berries and combine with other ingredients. Freeze. Spoon into sherbet glasses to serve.

Strawberry Mousse II

1 (8–ounce) package fat–free
  cream cheese
1¼ cups Domino strawberry
  flavored confectioners sugar

2 cups Dream Whip, prepared
  (see page 329), or Cool Whip
  Free

With a mixer, beat cream cheese until smooth. Add sugar; beat well. Fold in Dream Whip or Cool Whip Free.

Candied Orange Peel

Orange peel from 4 oranges
1 cup sugar
½ cup water

Dash salt
Confectioners sugar for coating

Wash oranges. Remove peel and cut in narrow strips. Boil in salted water for 15 minutes. Drain and cover with water again; bring to a boil. Drain. Combine sugar and water and bring to a boil, stirring to dissolve sugar. Add peel and cook until syrup is almost gone. Remove peels with a slotted spoon and place on waxed paper. Roll in sugar.

Cherry–Vanilla Fudge

2 cups sugar
1 cup skim milk
½ teaspoon salt
1 tablespoon Ultra Promise
   70% Less Fat

1 teaspoon vanilla extract
½ cup marshmallow creme
½ cup chopped candied
   cherries
2 to 3 drops red food coloring

In a heavy saucepan, combine sugar, milk and salt. Heat over medium heat, stirring constantly until sugar dissolves and mixture comes to a boil. Cook to soft ball stage (238°), stirring occasionally. Remove from heat. Add Promise and food coloring. Cool to lukewarm or 110°, without stirring. Add vanilla. Beat vigorously until mixture begins to hold its shape. Add marshmallow creme; beat until fudge becomes very thick and loses its gloss. Quickly stir in cherries and spread on a Pam–sprayed platter. Cut into squares when firm but still slightly warm.

Peanut Butter Fudge

2 cups sugar
1 cup skim milk
2 tablespoons reduced–fat
   peanut butter

1½ tablespoons Ultra Promise
   70% Less Fat
1 teaspoon vanilla

Mix sugar and milk well. Add peanut butter. Heat to boiling and cook on slow boil until it reaches soft ball stage, stirring occasionally. Remove from heat and let rest and cool for 15 minutes. Add Ultra Promise and vanilla. Beat until it begins to lose its gloss. Pour onto Pam–sprayed platter and let sit until hardened. Cut into squares.

Angel Food Cake

1 cup cake flour
1½ cups sugar, divided
1½ cups egg whites
½ teaspoon salt

2½ tablespoons cold water
1½ teaspoons cream of tartar
1 teaspoon vanilla extract
½ teaspoon butter extract

Sift flour and ½ cup sugar together. Place egg whites in large bowl; add salt and water. Whip until frothy. Add cream of tartar; whip until mixture stands in stiff peaks. Whip in remaining sugar. Fold in a portion of the flour mixture; add vanilla and butter extracts. Add remaining flour mixture. Pour batter into ungreased angel food cake pan. Bake at 350° for 45 minutes.

Apple Yorkshire Cake

3 tablespoons Fleischmann's
Fat Free Squeezable Spread
3 tablespoons Ultra Promise
70% Less Fat
½ cup brown sugar
1½ teaspoons cinnamon

2½ cups apples, peeled, cored
and sliced
1½ cups flour
⅛ cup sugar
¾ teaspoon salt
3 Egg Beaters
1½ cups skim milk

Melt Promise and Fleischmann's in a 9 x 9–inch Pam–sprayed baking dish. Sprinkle brown sugar and cinnamon evenly over "butter". Arrange apples over sugar. In a separate bowl, combine remaining ingredients and beat until well blended. Carefully pour over apples. Bake at 450° for 23 minutes.

SYRUP:
1 cup water
1 cup sugar

¼ teaspoon vanilla extract

Bring to boil and cook 3 minutes. While cake is warm, poke holes with a knife and pour syrup over while cake and syrup are hot.

Applesauce Cake

1 package Butter Buds Liquid
   (see page 50)
1 cup sugar
1 teaspoon cinnamon
⅛ teaspoon cloves
½ teaspoon allspice
½ teaspoon nutmeg
½ teaspoon salt
2 cups self–rising flour
¼ cup skim milk
1 cup raisins
½ cup pineapple, crushed
1 cup applesauce

Mix together dry ingredients. Cream Butter Buds Liquid and sugar; add to dry ingredients. Add milk, raisins, pineapple and applesauce. Mix well. Pour into a Pam–sprayed 9 x 9–inch pan. Bake at 350° for 50 to 55 minutes. Cover top with aluminum if browning too much. Top with icing.

ICING:

1 tablespoon Ultra Promise
   70% Less Fat
⅓ cup powdered sugar
Drop of vanilla extract
Evaporated skimmed milk

Add Promise and sugar and mix to make a paste. Add enough milk to make spreadable; add vanilla. Spread on warm cake.

Apricot Coffee Cake

5 tablespoons Ultra Promise
   70% Less Fat
¾ cup Butter Buds Liquid
   (see page 50)
2 cups sugar
2 Egg Beaters
1 cup Fat Free sour cream
1 teaspoon almond extract
2 cups all–purpose flour
1 teaspoon baking powder
¼ teaspoon salt
1 (10–ounce) jar apricot
   preserves
½ cup brown sugar

Cream together Promise, Butter Buds Liquid and sugar. Add Egg Beaters and mix well. Fold in sour cream and extract. In a separate bowl sift together flour, baking powder and salt. Fold flour mixture into the sugar mixture. Put half of the cake batter in a Pam–sprayed tube pan. Top with preserves and brown sugar. Spoon remaining batter on top. Bake at 350° for 48 minutes or until done.

Baked Date "Pudding" Cake

¾ cup boiling water
1 cup pitted dates, diced
3 tablespoons Ultra Promise
  70% Less Fat
1 Egg Beater
½ cup brown sugar

½ cup orange marmalade
½ cup pineapple preserves
1¾ cups self–rising flour
1 teaspoon salt
Rebel Sauce (see page 81)

Pour water over dates; add Promise. Combine Egg Beater, brown sugar, marmalade and preserves. Stir into date mixture. Combine flour and salt. Stir into date mixture until just moist. Pour into a Pam–sprayed 9 x 13–inch pan. Bake at 350° for 28 minutes or until done. Serve with Rebel Sauce.

Butter Cake

5 tablespoons Ultra Promise
  70% Less Fat
3 tablespoons Fleischmann's
  Fat Free Squeezable Spread

½ cup Butter Buds Liquid
  (see page 50)
2 cups sugar
2 cups self–rising flour
5 Egg Beaters

Cream together Promise, Fleischmann's, Butter Buds Liquid and sugar. Add flour and Egg Beaters; mix well. Pour into a Pam–sprayed tube pan. Bake at 350° for 50 minutes or until done. Do not over bake.

Cherry Cake

1¼ cups sugar
2 tablespoons Ultra Promise
  70% Less Fat
1 Egg Beater

1 can drained cherries (sour)
1 cup self–rising flour
1 teaspoon cinnamon
½ teaspoon almond extract

Cut Promise into sugar; add Egg Beater and cherries and stir with a spoon. Add dry ingredients and almond extract. Bake at 375° for 40 minutes.

Cherry Pudding Cake with Sauce

1 cup sugar	1 Egg Beater
3 tablespoons Ultra Promise 70% Less Fat	1 cup self–rising flour
	1 can red sour cherries
1 tablespoon Fleischmann's Fat Free Squeezable Spread	Juice of cherries, divided

Mix together first 6 ingredients with ⅓ cup reserved juice. Mix well. Pour into a Pam–sprayed 9 x 9–inch pan. Bake at 350° for 22 minutes or until done.

SAUCE:

Remaining cherry juice	1 tablespoon flour
1 cup sugar	

Bring to boil and cook 2 minutes. Pour over pudding while warm.

Brandy Torte

2 cups Zwieback crumbs	1 tablespoon lemon rind
1½ cups pretzel crumbs	2 teaspoons vanilla extract
½ teaspoon cinnamon	4 Egg Beaters
½ teaspoon salt	6 egg whites
2 teaspoons baking powder	1 cup sugar

Mix first 6 ingredients. In separate bowl, add vanilla and Egg Beaters. Gradually add sugar, beating until well mixed. Add to dry ingredients; mix thoroughly. Beat egg whites until stiff; fold into mixture. Pour into a 9 x 13–inch Pam–sprayed casserole dish. Bake at 350° for 28 minutes. Meanwhile prepare Brandy Sauce.

BRANDY SAUCE:

2 cups water	2 tablespoons grated orange rind
1 cup sugar	
¼ cup brandy	2 tablespoons orange juice

Place water and sugar in saucepan; heat to boiling, stirring until sugar is dissolved. Continue cooking over medium high heat for 30 minutes or until syrupy. Add brandy and orange juice. Slowly pour syrup over hot torte until it is completely absorbed.

Banana Pound Cake with Sauce

3 large bananas
1 cup sugar
2 tablespoons Ultra Promise
   70% Less Fat
1½ Egg Beaters

½ teaspoon vanilla extract
1½ cups self–rising flour
¼ teaspoon salt
Banana Sauce (see page 70)

Mash bananas, add vanilla; set aside. Cream Promise and sugar. Add Egg Beaters and mix well. Stir in banana mixture alternately with flour and salt. Bake in a Pam–sprayed Bundt cake pan for 34 minutes. Punch holes in warm cake with toothpick. Top with Banana Sauce.

Blackberry Cake

1 bag blackberries, frozen
1¾ cups sugar
¼ cup corn syrup
½ cup Butter Buds Liquid
   (see page 50)
3 tablespoons Ultra Promise
   70% Less Fat

2 teaspoons cinnamon
2 teaspoons allspice
2 teaspoons nutmeg
3 cups self–rising flour
5 Egg Beaters

Blend blackberries in blender; set aside. Mix sugar, corn syrup, Butter Buds Liquid, Promise, spices and Egg Beaters. Add alternately the blackberries and flour. Bake in a Pam–sprayed Bundt cake pan at 375° for 40 minutes. May be iced with a sugar glaze.

Chocolate Angel Food Cake

11 large egg whites
1 teaspoon cream of tartar
½ teaspoon salt
1 teaspoon vanilla extract

1½ cups sugar
¾ cup cake flour
¼ cup cocoa

Sift together sugar, flour and cocoa. Beat egg whites with cream of tartar and salt until very stiff. Gradually fold flour mixture into egg mixture. Add flavoring while folding in flour mixture. Pour into a tube pan. Bake in a cold oven set at 325° for 45 minutes or until done.

Chocolate Cake

1 cup self–rising flour
1 cup sugar
¼ teaspoon salt
1 Egg Beater
½ teaspoon soda
¼ cup non–fat buttermilk
½ teaspoon vanilla extract

¼ cup Ultra Promise 70% Less
  Fat
¼ cup Fleischmann's Fat Free
  Squeezable Spread
½ cup water
1½ tablespoons cocoa

Mix together flour, sugar and salt; set aside. In a separate bowl, mix Egg Beater, soda, buttermilk and vanilla; set aside. In a small saucepan, add Promise, Fleischmann's, water and cocoa; bring to a boil and pour over flour mixture. Stir. Add buttermilk mixture and mix well. Pour into a Pam–sprayed 12 x 7½–inch baking dish. Bake at 350° for 18 minutes.

Chocolate Pudding Cake

¾ cup sugar
1 cup self–rising flour
2 tablespoons cocoa
1½ cups skim milk
3 tablespoons Karo

1 tablespoon Butter Buds
  powder
1 teaspoon vanilla extract
1½ cups water

TOPPING:
½ cup sugar
½ cup brown sugar

¼ cup cocoa

Mix cake ingredients and pour into a deep Pam–sprayed casserole dish. Mix topping and sprinkle over cake. Pour 1½ cups water over top. DO NOT STIR. Bake at 350° for 45 minutes. Serve while hot, a la mode.

Devil's Food

1½ cups self–rising flour
1½ cups sugar
½ cup cocoa
¼ teaspoon cream of tartar
2 tablespoons Ultra Promise
   70% Less Fat

3 tablespoons Fleischmann's
   Fat Free Squeezable Spread
1 cup skim milk
1 teaspoon vanilla extract
½ cup Egg Beaters

Mix together all dry ingredients; add Promise, Fleischmann's and ¾ cup milk. Beat on medium for 2 minutes. Add ¼ cup milk, vanilla and Egg Beaters. Beat an additional 2 minutes. Pour into 2 Pam–sprayed cake pans or sheet pan. Bake at 350° for 21 minutes.

Hot Milk Cake

1 cup self–rising flour
¼ teaspoon salt
2 tablespoons Ultra Promise
   70% Less Fat

½ cup skim milk, scalded
2 Egg Beaters
1 cup sugar
1 teaspoon vanilla extract

Mix together flour and salt; set aside. Mix together Promise, milk and extract; keep hot. Beat together Egg Beaters and sugar. Add dry ingredients to egg mixture, stirring just until blended. Stir in hot milk mixture. Bake in a Pam–sprayed loaf pan at 350° for 18 minutes. Reduce heat to 300° for 7 minutes or until done.

Lemon Supreme Cake

1 box Better Crocker Lemon Fat
   Free Sweet Rewards cake mix

Lemon Glaze (see page 332)

Prepare cake according to directions. Prepare glaze. Pour glaze on warm cake.

Iced Cocktail Cake

1½ cups sugar
2 Egg Beaters

2 cups self–rising flour
1 (1–pound) can fruit cocktail

Beat Egg Beaters and sugar together. Alternate flour and juice from fruit cocktail to egg mixture. Fold in fruit last. Pour into Pam–sprayed sheet cake pan.

ICING:
¾ cup sugar
½ cup evaporated skimmed
  milk
¼ cup Ultra Promise 70% Less
  Fat

¼ cup Butter Buds Liquid
  (see page 50)
1 teaspoon vanilla extract

Blend all ingredients in a saucepan. Boil for 10 minutes. Spoon hot onto warm cake. Good warm or cold.

Orange Sponge Cake

1 cup Egg Beaters
1 tablespoon orange peel
½ cup orange juice
1½ cups sugar, divided
1 teaspoon orange extract

¼ teaspoon salt
1⅓ cups cake flour
6 egg whites
1 teaspoon cream of tartar
Orange Frosting (see page 331)

Mix together Egg Beaters, orange peel and juice. Add 1 cup sugar, extract and salt. Fold in flour. Beat egg whites until foamy. Add cream of tartar; beat until soft peaks form. Gradually add ½ cup sugar, beating until stiff peaks form. Thoroughly fold whites into batter. Bake in Pam–sprayed 10–inch tube pan at 325° for 45 minutes or until done. May be iced with Orange Frosting. Also good with Lemon Sauce (see page 76).

Mincemeat Cake

1½ cups Kellogg's All–Bran
  cereal
1¼ cups skim milk
1¼ cups self–rising flour
½ cup sugar

1 Egg Beater
¼ cup Ultra Promise 70% Less
  Fat
1 cup mincemeat
1 can fat–free Eagle Brand milk

Mix together cereal and milk; set aside until cereal is softened. Stir together flour and sugar; set aside. Mix together Egg Beater and Promise. Add this to cereal mixture, stirring well. Add flour mixture, stirring only until combined. Add mincemeat. Fold in Eagle Brand milk. Bake at 350° for 35 minutes or until done.

Praline Cake

1½ cups self–rising flour
1½ cups brown sugar
¾ cup skim milk
¼ cup Ultra Promise 70% Less
  Fat

¼ cup Fleischmann's Fat Free
  Squeezable Spread
2 Egg Beaters
2 teaspoons vanilla extract
½ recipe Caramel Icing
  (see page 328)

Measure all ingredients in a mixing bowl and beat with an electric mixer for 3 minutes on high. Pour into Pam–sprayed Bundt pan. Bake at 350° for 40 minutes. Meanwhile, prepare ½ of the Caramel Icing. Ice cake while warm.

Quick Coffee Cake

2 cups Pioneer lowfat biscuit
  mix
4 Egg Beaters

1 box light brown sugar
1 teaspoon vanilla extract

Combine all ingredients. Pour into 9 x 12–inch Pam–sprayed pan. Bake at 350° for 30 minutes. Sprinkle with confectioners sugar while warm. Top with sliced fruit of your choice.

Petit Fours

White Layer Cake (see page 318)   Strawberry Icing (see page 331)

Prepare cake as directed; let cool. Cut cake into small servings or desired shapes, about 2–inch square in size. Set aside.

Prepare Strawberry Icing as directed. Spoon mixture over cakes and decorate as desired.

VARIATIONS: Lemon Icing and Chocolate Icing may be used in place of Strawberry.

Prune Cake

2 cups flour
2 cups sugar
1 teaspoon cinnamon
1 teaspoon nutmeg
1 teaspoon allspice
1 teaspoon soda
½ teaspoon salt
3 Egg Beaters

1 cup non–fat buttermilk
6 tablespoons Ultra Promise
   70% Less Fat
½ cup Butter Buds Liquid
   (see page 50)
1 cup baby food prunes
Vanilla Icing (see page 331)

Sift together dry ingredients. Mix together buttermilk, Promise, Butter Buds Liquid and prunes. Stir in Egg Beaters. Pour into dry mixture; stir well. Pour into a Pam–sprayed Bundt pan. Bake at 350° for 30 to 35 minutes or until done to the touch. Ice cooled cake with icing.

Red Devil's Food

4 tablespoons Ultra Promise
  70% Less Fat
¼ cup Butter Buds Liquid
  (see page 50)
1 cup sugar
1 teaspoon salt
1 teaspoon vanilla extract
⅓ cup cold water

½ cup cocoa
2½ cups cake flour
1 cup cold water
3 egg whites
¾ cup sugar
1½ teaspoons soda
⅓ cup water

Blend together first 3 ingredients. Add salt, vanilla and cocoa. Beat ⅓ cup cold water into sugar mixture. Add flour alternately with 1 cup cold water, beating after each addition. Beat egg whites until soft peaks form. Gradually add ¾ cup sugar, beating until stiff. Fold into batter. Dissolve soda in ⅓ cup water; stir into batter, mixing thoroughly. Bake in a Pam–sprayed 9 x 13–inch pan at 350° for 30 minutes.

Red Velvet Cake

4 tablespoons Ultra Promise
  70% Less Fat
½ cup Butter Buds Liquid
  (see page 50)
2 cups sugar
2 Egg Beaters
2 ounces red food coloring
2 tablespoons cocoa

1 teaspoon vanilla extract
1 cup non–fat buttermilk
1 teaspoon salt
2½ cups cake flour
1 tablespoon vinegar
¾ teaspoon soda
Frosting (see page 328–331)

Cream together first 3 ingredients. Add Egg Beaters, one at a time, beating thoroughly after each addition. Add vanilla, flour, buttermilk, alternately. Add coloring and cocoa. Add salt, vinegar and soda. Mix with batter. Pour into two 9–inch Pam–sprayed cake pans. Bake at 350° for 23 minutes. Split layers and frost.

Spice Layer Cake

4 tablespoons Ultra Promise
  70% Less Fat
½ cup Butter Buds Liquid
  (see page 50)
1 cup sugar
2¼ cups cake flour
1 teaspoon baking powder
1 teaspoon salt
¾ teaspoon soda

1 teaspoon cinnamon
¾ teaspoon cloves
¾ cup brown sugar
1 cup non–fat buttermilk
3 Egg Beaters
Date Filling (see page 329)
Brown Sugar Frosting
  (see page 328)

Combine flour, sugar, baking powder, salt, soda and spices. Add brown sugar and buttermilk, stirring until all flour is dampened. Add Egg Beaters, Promise and Butter Buds Liquid. Beat thoroughly. Bake in Pam–sprayed 9–inch round pans at 350° for 25 minutes.

To complete cake, place Date Filling between layers and ice with Brown Sugar Frosting.

Sponge Cake

4 Egg Beaters
6 egg whites
1½ cups sugar
1 teaspoon vanilla extract

1¼ cups self–rising flour
½ teaspoon salt
¼ cup cold water

Beat together Egg Beaters, sugar and vanilla. Add flour and salt alternately to egg mixture with cold water. In separate bowl, beat egg whites until stiff, but not dry. Fold egg whites into batter. Pour into Pam–sprayed angel food pan. Bake at 325° for 43 minutes. Cover with aluminum foil after 15 to 18 minutes to prevent over browning. Cool for 10 minutes before inverting onto cake plate.

Texas Sheet Cake

1 cup self–rising flour
1 cup sugar
¼ cup fat–free sour cream
½ teaspoon vanilla extract
1 package Butter Buds powder

2 tablespoons Ultra Promise
  70% Less Fat
½ cup water
1 Egg Beater

Combine flour and sugar; set aside. In a small saucepan, combine sour cream, vanilla, Butter Buds, Promise and water. Bring mixture to a boil, remove from heat and blend with flour mixture. Stir in Egg Beaters. Pour into a 9 x 9–inch Pam–sprayed pan. Bake at 350° for 28 minutes.

Vanilla Cake

4 tablespoons Ultra Promise
  70% Less Fat
½ cup Butter Buds Liquid
  (see page 50)
2 cups sugar
1 teaspoon vanilla extract
¼ teaspoon lemon extract

¼ teaspoon butter extract
2½ cups cake flour
3 teaspoons baking powder
¾ teaspoon salt
½ cup skim milk
½ cup water
6 egg whites

Cream together first 3 ingredients. Add extracts. Combine dry ingredients; add to creamed mixture alternately with milk and water. Beat after each addition. Beat egg whites until stiff. Fold in egg whites. Pour into two 9–inch Pam–sprayed pie pans. Bake at 350° for 23 minutes. When thoroughly cooled, cut each layer in half, making a total of 4 layers.

White Layer Cake

4 tablespoons Ultra Promise
  70% Less Fat
3/8 cup Butter Buds Liquid
  (see page 50)
1½ teaspoons vanilla extract
1½ cups sugar

2½ cups cake flour
1½ teaspoons baking powder
½ teaspoon salt
1⅓ cups nonfat buttermilk
4 egg whites

Cream together Promise, Butter Buds Liquid, vanilla and all but ¼ cup sugar. Sift together dry ingredients; add to creamed mixture alternately with buttermilk, starting and ending with dry ingredients. Beat egg whites until foamy. Gradually add the remaining ¼ cup of sugar. Beat to stiff peaks. Fold into batter. Pour into two 9–inch Pam–sprayed cake pans and bake at 350° for 25 minutes or one 9 x 13–inch Pam–sprayed cake pan and cook for 33 minutes. DO NOT OVER COOK.

Boiled Custard Ice Cream

5½ cups skim milk
2 cups sugar
9 Egg Beaters
1 (16–ounce) carton Land O
  Lakes Fat Free Half & Half

3 (12–ounce) cans evaporated
  skimmed milk
1 tablespoon vanilla extract
½ teaspoon salt

Scald skim milk. Remove from heat. Slowly stir in sugar and Egg Beaters. Reheat and cook until wooden spoon is well coated. Add Half & Half, evaporated skimmed milk, vanilla, and salt. Remove and set in pan of cold water until cool. Pour into ice cream freezer and process.

NOTE: You may add extra milk after cooking if needed for 6 quart freezer.

Blueberry Sorbet

2¼ cups ripe blueberries,
  washed and drained

½ cup pineapple juice
¼ cup honey

Combine all ingredients in container of electric blender; process until smooth. Pour mixture into an 8–inch square freezable container. Cover and freeze until firm. To serve, spoon into individual dessert dishes.

Homemade Banana Ice Cream

6 Egg Beaters
1½ cups sugar
2 teaspoons vanilla extract

2 cans fat–free Eagle Brand
  milk
½ gallon skim milk
6 bananas

Mix Egg Beaters and sugar. Add vanilla extract and Eagle Brand milk. Stir well. Add skim milk and bananas. Mix well. Turn into electric ice cream freezer and process until frozen.

VARIATION: Substitute 3 cups of fresh peaches in place of bananas.

Honeydew Melon Frost

3 cups honeydew melon, cubed
¼ cup Triple Sec

3 tablespoons lemon juice
2½ tablespoons sugar

Combine ingredients in container of an electric blender; process until smooth. Pour mixture into an 8–inch square freezable pan. Cover and freeze until firm. To serve, spoon frozen mixture into individual dessert dishes. May be garnished with a lemon slice.

VARIATION: Substitute cantaloupe in place of honeydew melon.

Orange Sorbet

1 (3–ounce) package orange
   gelatin
1 cup boiling water
1 cup cold water
¾ cup light corn syrup

2 Egg Beaters
1 tablespoon orange juice
1 tablespoon orange rind,
   grated

Dissolve gelatin in boiling water. Stir in cold water and corn syrup. Beat in Egg Beaters, orange juice and rind, using a wire whisk. Pour into a freezable 9 x 13–inch dish. Cover and freeze for 2 hours. Spoon half of mixture into blender and process for about 25 seconds. Repeat with remaining ingredients. Pour into a 1½–quart container. Cover and freeze overnight.

VARIATION: For lime sorbet, substitute lime gelatin, lime juice and lime rind in place of orange gelatin, orange juice and orange rind.

Strawberry Sherbet

1 envelope unflavored gelatin
1 cup orange juice
Grated orange peel
Grated peel and juice of 1
   lemon

¼ cup sugar
1½ cups strawberries, mashed
½ cup applesauce

In saucepan, soften gelatin in orange and lemon juice. Add sugar and peels. Stir over low heat until gelatin and sugar are dissolved. Cool. Stir in strawberries and applesauce. Pour into shallow pan. Freeze until firm.

Biscotti

4 cups all–purpose flour
2½ tablespoons baking powder
½ teaspoon salt
⅓ cup Ultra Promise 70% Less
    Fat

6 Egg Beaters
1 cup sugar
3 teaspoons vanilla, orange,
    lemon or almond extract

Sift together first 3 ingredients into a large mixing bowl. Cut Promise into flour mixture. In a separate bowl, mix together remaining ingredients. Combine with flour mixture; blend well. Knead dough on a lightly floured surface until smooth. Shape dough into 2 oblong loaves, ¾–inch thick. Place on 2 Pam–sprayed cookie sheets. Bake at 350° for 20 minutes. Cut into slices approximately ¾–inch thick. Place slices, cut side up, on cookie sheets and bake 5 minutes per side, until crisp and golden.

Butterscotch Goodies

2 tablespoons Peter Pan 30%
    less fat peanut butter
6 tablespoons Smucker's Fat
    Free Topping, butterscotch

4 cups corn flakes
Confectioners sugar

Heat peanut butter and butterscotch topping. Stir in corn flakes until well coated. Prepare baking sheet by lining with aluminum foil, then spray with Pam. Spoon mixture onto prepared pan. Place in a 300° oven and bake for 4 to 5 minutes. Remove from oven and let cool on pan. Sprinkle with confectioners sugar. Makes 12.

NOTE: May be sticky. Sprinkle with extra confectioners sugar.

Oatmeal Cookies

3 tablespoons Ultra Promise
    70% Less Fat
5 tablespoons Fleischmann's
    Fat Free Squeezable Spread
1 Egg Beater
1 cup flour

1 cup sugar
½ cup packed brown sugar
1 teaspoon vanilla extract
1¼ cups quick cooking rolled
    oatmeal

Mix together first 7 ingredients; blend well. Stir in oats. Drop dough on a Pam–sprayed cookie sheet 2 inches apart. Bake at 375° for 8 to 10 minutes depending on soft or crunchiness desired. Makes 40 cookies.

Lady Finger Treats

Day old fat–free white bread
Fat–free Eagle Brand milk

Brown sugar

Trim crust away from edges of bread. Cut into 3 lady finger slices. Brush liberally with Eagle Brand milk. Sprinkle with brown sugar. Bake at 350° until golden and bubbly.

Mincemeat Bars

1 (14–ounce) package oat bran
    muffin mix
1 cup mincemeat

1 (14–ounce) can fat–free Eagle
    Brand milk
1 cup confectioners sugar
1½ to 2 tablespoons skim milk

Combine first 3 ingredients. Spread evenly in a Pam–sprayed 9 x 13–inch baking dish. (Wet the back of a spoon to smooth dough). Bake at 350° for 25 minutes. Cool slightly. Meanwhile, mix sugar and skim milk. Drizzle over all.

Lace Cookies

2 egg whites, room temperature
⅓ cup sugar

½ teaspoon orange extract

Beat egg whites until soft peaks form. Gradually add sugar, 1 tablespoon at a time, beating until stiff peaks form. Fold in extract. Drop by teaspoons 1 inch apart onto waxed paper lined cookie sheets. Bake at 300° for 35 minutes. Cool slightly; remove gently from waxed paper. Cool completely on wire racks.

VARIATION: Coconut or lemon extract could be used instead of orange extract.

NOTE: Do not prepare this recipe on humid days.

Cookies

2 cups flour
½ cup Ultra Promise 70% Less Fat

½ cup confectioners sugar
½ cup sugar

Sift flour and sugars into a food processor container. Add Promise. Process just until well blended. Do not over process or dough will begin to form balls and become hard. With your hands, form a ball and wrap in plastic wrap; refrigerate until cool. Remove from refrigerator and roll out. Cut with a 2–inch biscuit cutter.

VARIATIONS: Cinnamon–Raisin: Place three raisins in each cookie. Sprinkle with cinnamon–sugar and bake at 325° for 6 to 9 minutes.

Fruit filled: With your thumb, make an imprint in each cookie. Fill each cavity with a small amount of jam or preserves of your choice. Bake at 325° for 6 to 9 minutes.

Peanut Butter Surprise Cookies

1¾ cups all–purpose flour
1 teaspoon baking powder
⅛ teaspoon baking soda
½ cup Fleischmann's Fat Free
  Squeezable Spread
½ cup reduced fat peanut
  butter

1 cup sugar
½ cup brown sugar, packed
1 Egg Beater
1 teaspoon vanilla extract
Sugar
Milky Way Lites, miniatures,
  cut in half

Mix flour, baking powder and soda. Set aside. In separate bowl, beat together Fleischmann's and peanut butter. Add sugars and beat until fluffy. Add Egg Beater and vanilla. Beat until thoroughly combined. Add flour mixture. Dip out into 1–inch balls onto a Pam–sprayed cookie sheet. Sprinkle with sugar. Bake in 350° oven for 8 to 10 minutes. Immediately press ½ of Milky Way Lite miniatures, cut side down, in hot cookie.

So Easy Lemon Cookies

2⅔ cups Pioneer Low–fat
  Biscuit Mix
2 cups Domino lemon flavored
  confectioners sugar

1 teaspoon ground cinnamon
2 Egg Beaters
¼ cup skim milk
1 teaspoon vanilla extract

In a large bowl, combine biscuit mix, sugar and cinnamon. Add Egg Beaters, milk and extract. Stir well. Drop by teaspoonfuls, 2 inches apart, onto a Pam–sprayed cookie sheet. Bake at 350° for 8 to 10 minutes for softer cookies or 10 to 12 minutes for firmer cookies. Sprinkle with lemon flavored confectioners sugar or frost with Lemon Icing (see page 330).

Skillet Cookies

2 tablespoons Ultra Promise
  70% Less Fat
1 cup pitted dates, finely diced
1 cup sugar

2 Egg Beaters
3½ cups Rice Krispies
Confectioners sugar

Melt Promise in non–stick skillet; add dates, granulated sugar and Egg Beaters. Cook over low heat, stirring constantly until mixture forms a ball when dropped in cold water. Remove from heat; cool slightly. Stir in Rice Krispies, mixing well. Spoon out on a piece of waxed paper. Roll in confectioners sugar.

So Easy Chocolate Cookies

2⅔ cups Pioneer Low–fat
  Biscuit Mix
2 cups Domino chocolate
  flavored confectioners sugar

2 Egg Beaters
¼ cup skim milk
1 teaspoon vanilla extract

In a large bowl, combine biscuit mix and sugar. Add Egg Beaters, milk and extract. Stir well. Drop by teaspoonfuls, 2 inches apart, onto a Pam–sprayed cookie sheet. Bake at 350° for 8 to 10 minutes for softer cookies or 10 to 12 minutes for firmer cookies.

So Easy Strawberry Cookies

2⅔ cups Pioneer Low–fat
  Biscuit Mix
2 cups Domino strawberry
  flavored confectioners sugar

1 teaspoon ground cinnamon
2 Egg Beaters
¼ cup skim milk
1 teaspoon vanilla extract

In a large bowl, combine biscuit mix, sugar and cinnamon. Add Egg Beaters, milk and extract. Stir well. Drop by teaspoonfuls, 2 inches apart, onto a Pam–sprayed cookie sheet. Bake at 350° for 8 to 10 minutes for softer cookies or 10 to 12 minutes for firmer cookies. Sprinkle with strawberry flavored confectioners sugar or frost with Strawberry Icing (see page 331).

Graham Cracker Crust

1 cup Graham cracker crumbs
¼ cup sugar

3½ tablespoons fat–free sour
cream

Combine all ingredients well. Press into a Pam–sprayed pie pan.
May be cooked at 400° for 7 to 8 minutes or as is.

Chocolate Crust

1⅓ cups Pioneer Low–fat
Biscuit Mix
1 cup Domino chocolate
flavored confectioners sugar

1 Egg Beater
¼ cup skim milk
1 teaspoon vanilla extract

Combine all ingredients into a food processor. Process until crumbly
Press into a 9–inch Pam–sprayed pie plate. Bake at 350° for 5 minutes. Let cool completely before using.

Dessert Pie Shell

2 cups self–rising flour
⅛ cup sugar
3 tablespoons Weight
Watcher's Fat Free Whipped
Dressing
1 tablespoon fat-free sour
cream

¼ cup Ultra Promise 70% Less
Fat
1 tablespoon Fleischmann's Fat
Free Squeezable Spread
6 tablespoons ice water

Mix together flour and sugar. Cut in whipped dressing and Promise.
Add sour cream and Fleischmann's, mixing well. Add water. Mix
until dough lets go of side of bowl. Knead on floured bowl only until
desired consistency. Divide in half. Roll out, thinly. Line pie plate.
Cut sides and pinch dough together on pie plate lip. If recipe calls for
a cooked crust, pierce bottom and sides with a fork. Bake at 400° for
6 minutes or until golden. Makes two 9–inch pie shells.

Meringue Shell

3 egg whites   Scant of salt
3 tablespoons sugar

In a medium mixing bowl add egg whites and salt; beat until frothy. Add sugar one tablespoon at a time, beating well after each tablespoon. Beat until stiff peaks form. Spread meringue over entire area, touching pie shell or edge of dish. Bake at 350° for 10 minutes or until golden.

Fat Free Pie Shell

2 cups self–rising flour   1 tablespoon fat–free sour
⅛ cup sugar   cream
3 tablespoons Weight   3 tablespoons Fleischmann's
  Watcher's Fat Free Whipped   Fat Free Squeezable Spread
  Dressing   6 to 7 tablespoons water

Mix together first 5 ingredients, mixing well. Add water. Mix until dough lets go of side of bowl. Lightly knead on a floured board until dough is of good consistency. Roll out as thin as possible. Line pie plate with dough. Pinch sides. If needed, pierce bottom and side with a fork. Cook at 400° for 5 minutes or until golden brown. Makes two 9–inch pie shells.

Top Pie Crust

½ cup flour   3 tablespoons ice water
½ tablespoon sugar   I Can't Believe It's Not Butter
½ tablespoon corn oil   spray

Combine first 3 ingredients and work until the consistency of cornmeal. Add water, stirring until dough pulls away from bowl. Lightly knead on floured board. Cut, using top of pie pan for right size. When top is adjusted, lightly spray with "I Can't Believe It's Not Butter" spray. Cook according to recipe's directions.

Pie Shell for Fruit Fillings

1 cup all–purpose flour
¾ teaspoon salt

¼ cup Ultra Promise 70% Less Fat
⅝ cup fat–free sour cream

Mix together flour and salt. Cut in Promise. Add sour cream and mix until well blended. Cover and chill dough 30 minutes before using. Lightly knead on floured surface; roll out. Use as is or cook at 400° for 12 to 15 minutes or until golden, depending on individual recipe.

Brown Sugar Frosting

2 unbeaten egg whites
¾ cup sugar
¾ cup brown sugar
¼ teaspoon cream of tartar

⅓ cup cold water
Dash of salt
1 teaspoon vanilla extract
¼ teaspoon butter extract

Place all ingredients, except extracts, in top of double boiler. Beat to blend. Place over boiling water and cook, beating constantly until frosting forms stiff peaks, about 7 minutes. Remove from stove. Add extracts and beat for 2 additional minutes.

Caramel Icing

¼ cup evaporated skimmed milk
½ cup light brown sugar
¼ cup Ultra Promise 70% Less Fat

2 cups confectioners sugar
1 teaspoon vanilla
Dash of salt

Boil milk, brown sugar and Ultra Promise for 1 minute, stirring constantly. Remove from heat. Add confectioners sugar; beat until smooth. Add vanilla. Ice warm cake.

Chocolate Icing

1 (16–ounce) box Domino
  chocolate flavored
  confectioners sugar

6 tablespoons skim milk

Mix sugar and milk together well. Great for icing, brushing or dipping over your favorite cakes, cookies or muffins.

Date Filling

1 (8–ounce) package chopped
  dates
½ cup orange juice

1 tablespoon brown sugar
1 teaspoon orange peel, grated

Combine ingredients in small saucepan and cook until thick, 2 to 3 minutes.

Devonshire Clotted Cream

3 ounces fat–free cream cheese
1 teaspoon confectioners sugar

1½ cups Dream Whip, prepared
  (see below), or Cool Whip
  Free

Bring cream cheese to room temperature. With a fork, mix in sugar until well blended. Fold Dream Whip or Cool Whip Free into mixture.

Dream Whip, Prepared

1 envelope Dream Whip
  whipped topping mix

½ cup skim milk
½ teaspoon vanilla extract

Mix all ingredients in a deep narrow–bottom bowl. Beat at high speed of electric mixer about 4 minutes, or until topping thickens and forms soft peaks. Makes about 2 cups.

Lemon Icing

1 (16–ounce) box Domino
lemon flavored confectioners
sugar

6 tablespoons skim milk

Mix sugar and milk together well. Great for icing, brushing or dripping over your favorite cakes, cookies or muffins.

Fluffy White Icing

3 egg whites
1½ cups sugar
5 tablespoons cold water

¼ teaspoon cream of tartar
1 teaspoon vanilla

Place first 4 ingredients in top of double boiler over rapidly boiling water. Beat with electric mixer for 7 minutes. Remove from heat and add vanilla. Beat well. Spread on cooled cake.

Fruit Filling

1 can fat–free Eagle Brand milk
1½ cups confectioners sugar,
sifted
1 teaspoon ground allspice

1 teaspoon cinnamon
¼ teaspoon cloves
1½ cups raisins, ground

Cook 5 minutes in top of double boiler. Cool.

Milk Chocolate Icing

1 package Butter Buds Powder
3 cups confectioners sugar
¼ cup + 1 tablespoon
evaporated skimmed milk

1 tablespoon cocoa
1 teaspoon vanilla extract

Cream all ingredients until smooth. For best results, heat for 15 to 20 seconds in the microwave until it is the consistency suitable for spreading. DO NOT BOIL.

Orange Frosting

½ cup orange marmalade
1 egg white

¾ cup sugar
Dash of salt

Combine all ingredients in top of double boiler. Cook over hot water, beating constantly with mixer for 3 to 4 minutes. Remove from heat; beat until mixture stands in peaks.

Strawberry Icing

1 (16–ounce) box Domino
   strawberry flavored
   confectioners sugar

6 tablespoons skim milk

Mix sugar and milk together well. Great for icing, brushing or dripping over your favorite cakes, cookies or muffins.

Vanilla Icing

2 cups sugar
1 teaspoon soda
6 tablespoons Ultra Promise
   70% Less Fat

1 cup nonfat buttermilk
Dash of salt
1 teaspoon vanilla extract

Combine all ingredients, except vanilla, in a saucepan. Cook over medium heat until mixture reaches the soft ball stage, stirring constantly. Remove from heat and add vanilla. Whip until icing thickens and loses its luster. Spread on cake.

Almond Glaze

½ cup confectioners sugar
1 teaspoon Fleischmann's Fat
   Free Squeezable Spread

½ teaspoon almond extract
Evaporated skimmed milk

Mix together first 3 ingredients. Add a small amount of milk to make desired consistency. Will glaze one loaf of bread or small coffee cake.

Lemon Glaze

1 cup confectioners sugar

Juice of 3 lemons

Combine and stir well.

Pineapple Glaze

3 tablespoons sugar
1 tablespoon cornstarch
1 cup pineapple juice

Dash of salt
¼ teaspoon orange peel, grated

Combine all ingredients in a small saucepan. Heat and stir to boiling. Let boil for 2 minutes. Use warm or at room temperature.

Vanilla Glaze

½ cup confectioners sugar
1 teaspoon Fleischmann's Fat
   Free Squeezable Spread

½ teaspoon vanilla extract
Skim milk

Mix together first 3 ingredients. Add a small amount of milk to make desired consistency. Will glaze one loaf of bread.

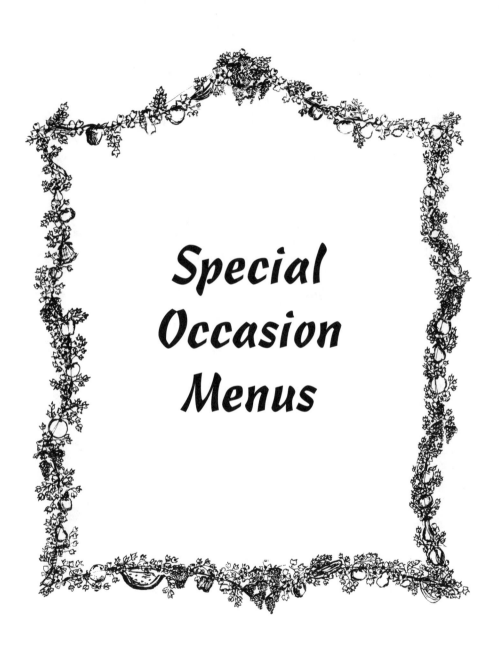

Special Occasion Menus

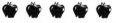

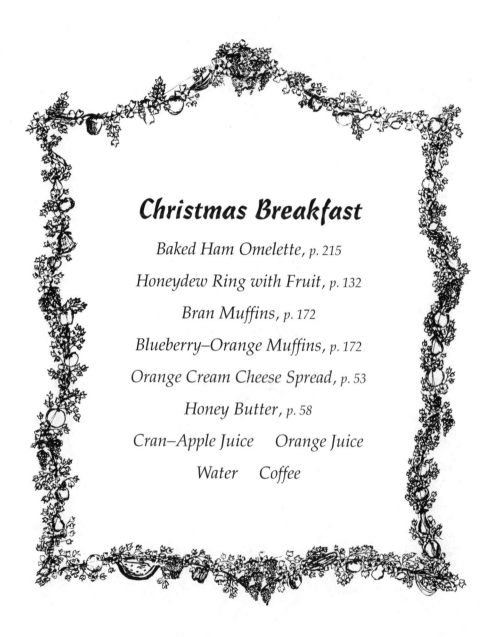

Christmas Breakfast

Baked Ham Omelette, p. 215

Honeydew Ring with Fruit, p. 132

Bran Muffins, p. 172

Blueberry–Orange Muffins, p. 172

Orange Cream Cheese Spread, p. 53

Honey Butter, p. 58

Cran–Apple Juice   Orange Juice

Water   Coffee

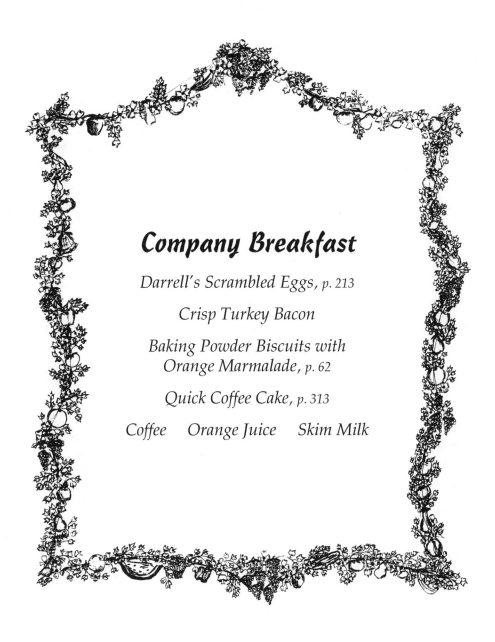

Company Breakfast

Darrell's Scrambled Eggs, p. 213

Crisp Turkey Bacon

*Baking Powder Biscuits with
Orange Marmalade,* p. 62

Quick Coffee Cake, p. 313

Coffee   Orange Juice   Skim Milk

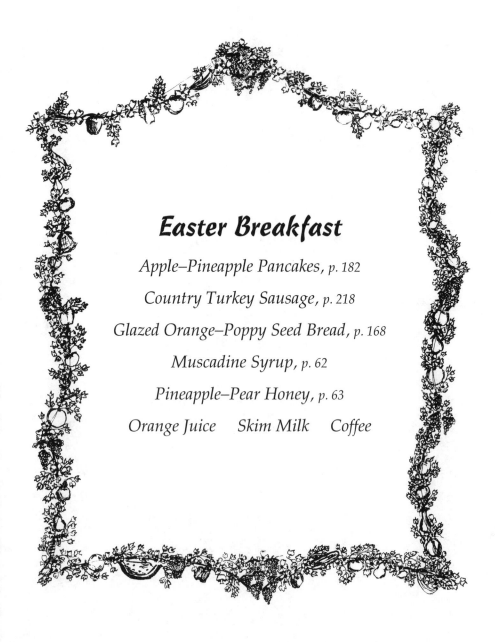

Easter Breakfast

Apple–Pineapple Pancakes, p. 182

Country Turkey Sausage, p. 218

Glazed Orange–Poppy Seed Bread, p. 168

Muscadine Syrup, p. 62

Pineapple–Pear Honey, p. 63

Orange Juice   Skim Milk   Coffee

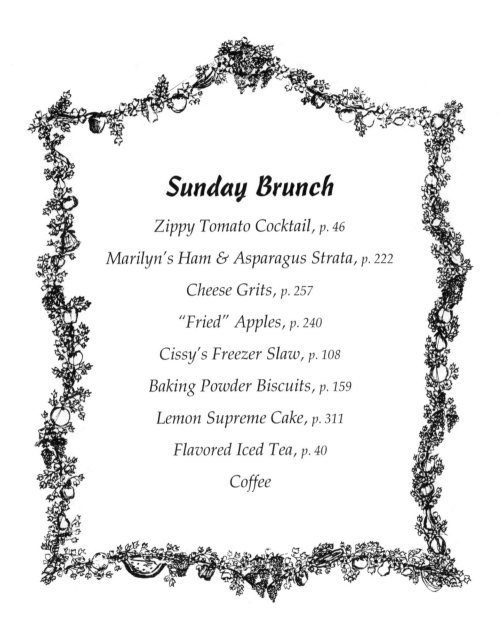

Sunday Brunch

Zippy Tomato Cocktail, p. 46

Marilyn's Ham & Asparagus Strata, p. 222

Cheese Grits, p. 257

"Fried" Apples, p. 240

Cissy's Freezer Slaw, p. 108

Baking Powder Biscuits, p. 159

Lemon Supreme Cake, p. 311

Flavored Iced Tea, p. 40

Coffee

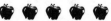

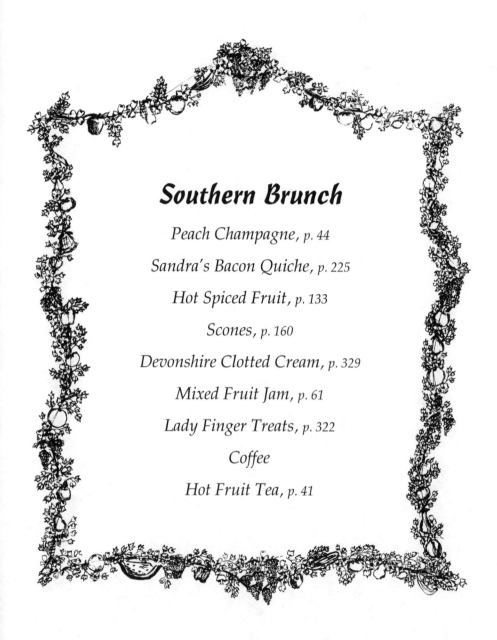

Southern Brunch

Peach Champagne, p. 44

Sandra's Bacon Quiche, p. 225

Hot Spiced Fruit, p. 133

Scones, p. 160

Devonshire Clotted Cream, p. 329

Mixed Fruit Jam, p. 61

Lady Finger Treats, p. 322

Coffee

Hot Fruit Tea, p. 41

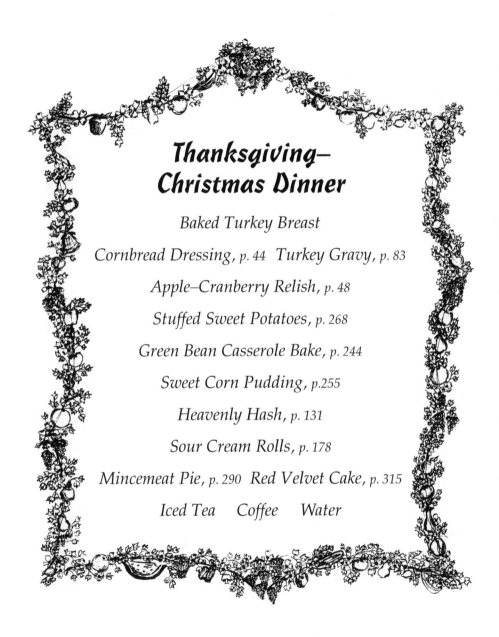

Thanksgiving– *Christmas Dinner*

Baked Turkey Breast

Cornbread Dressing, p. 44   *Turkey Gravy,* p. 83

Apple–Cranberry Relish, p. 48

Stuffed Sweet Potatoes, p. 268

Green Bean Casserole Bake, p. 244

Sweet Corn Pudding, p.255

Heavenly Hash, p. 131

Sour Cream Rolls, p. 178

Mincemeat Pie, p. 290   *Red Velvet Cake,* p. 315

Iced Tea   Coffee   Water

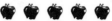
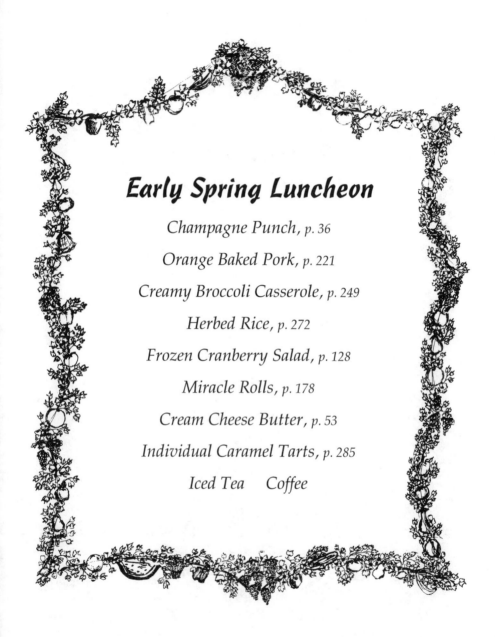

Early Spring Luncheon

Champagne Punch, p. 36

Orange Baked Pork, p. 221

Creamy Broccoli Casserole, p. 249

Herbed Rice, p. 272

Frozen Cranberry Salad, p. 128

Miracle Rolls, p. 178

Cream Cheese Butter, p. 53

Individual Caramel Tarts, p. 285

Iced Tea   Coffee

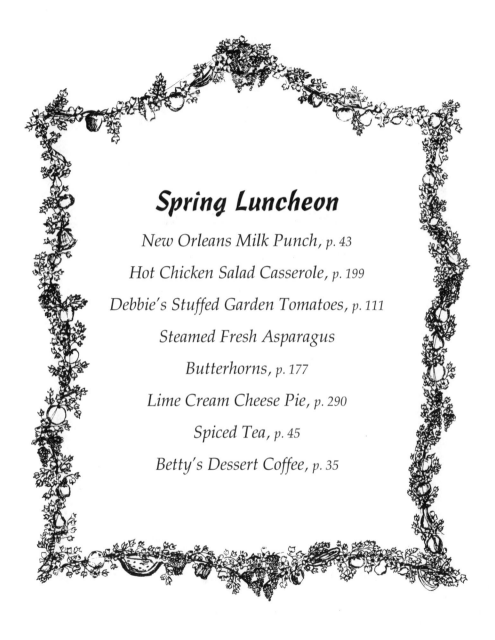

Spring Luncheon

New Orleans Milk Punch, p. 43

Hot Chicken Salad Casserole, p. 199

Debbie's Stuffed Garden Tomatoes, p. 111

Steamed Fresh Asparagus

Butterhorns, p. 177

Lime Cream Cheese Pie, p. 290

Spiced Tea, p. 45

Betty's Dessert Coffee, p. 35

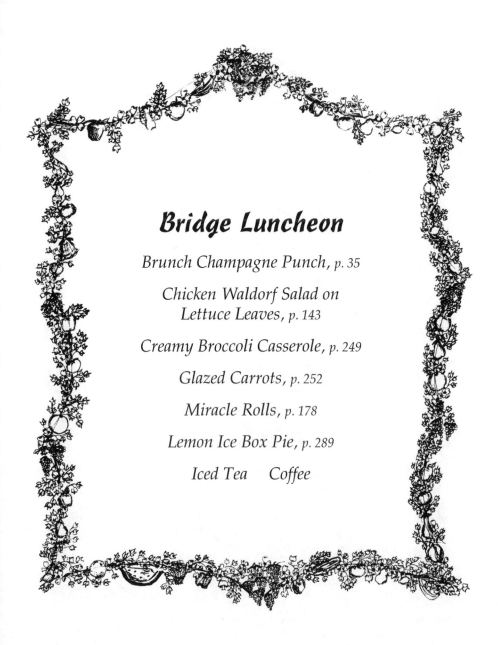

Bridge Luncheon

Brunch Champagne Punch, p. 35

Chicken Waldorf Salad on
Lettuce Leaves, p. 143

Creamy Broccoli Casserole, p. 249

Glazed Carrots, p. 252

Miracle Rolls, p. 178

Lemon Ice Box Pie, p. 289

Iced Tea   Coffee

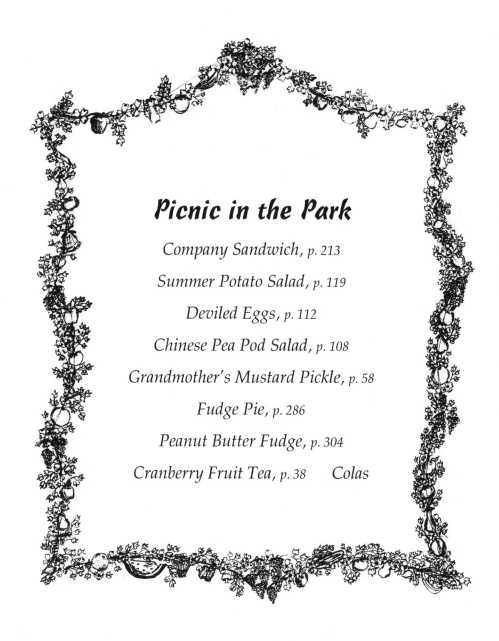

Picnic in the Park

Company Sandwich, p. 213

Summer Potato Salad, p. 119

Deviled Eggs, p. 112

Chinese Pea Pod Salad, p. 108

Grandmother's Mustard Pickle, p. 58

Fudge Pie, p. 286

Peanut Butter Fudge, p. 304

Cranberry Fruit Tea, p. 38   Colas

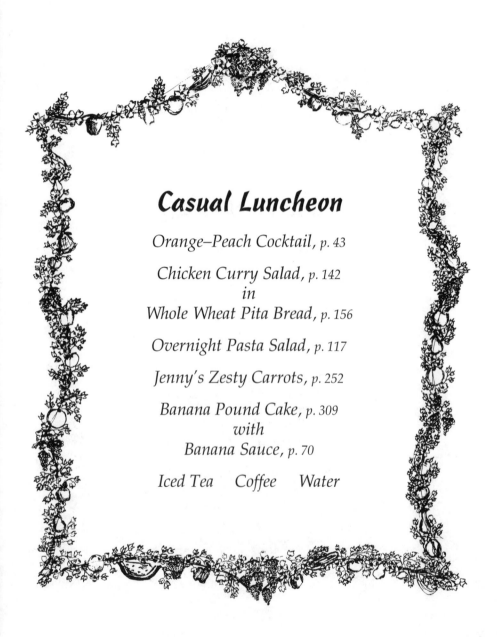

Casual Luncheon

Orange–Peach Cocktail, p. 43

Chicken Curry Salad, p. 142
in
Whole Wheat Pita Bread, p. 156

Overnight Pasta Salad, p. 117

Jenny's Zesty Carrots, p. 252

Banana Pound Cake, p. 309
with
Banana Sauce, p. 70

Iced Tea   Coffee   Water

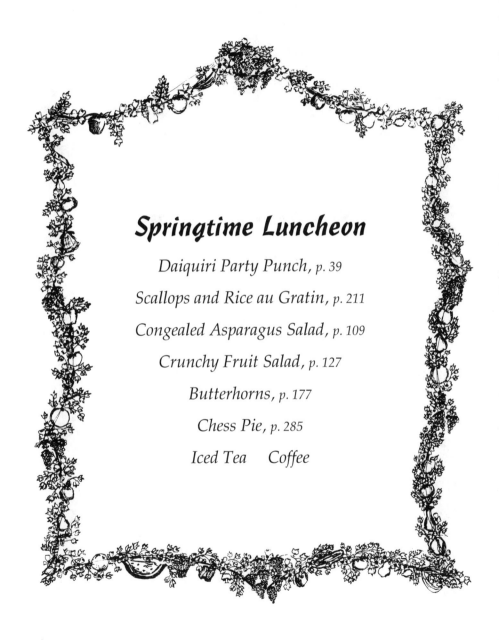

Springtime Luncheon

Daiquiri Party Punch, p. 39

Scallops and Rice au Gratin, p. 211

Congealed Asparagus Salad, p. 109

Crunchy Fruit Salad, p. 127

Butterhorns, p. 177

Chess Pie, p. 285

Iced Tea   Coffee

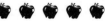

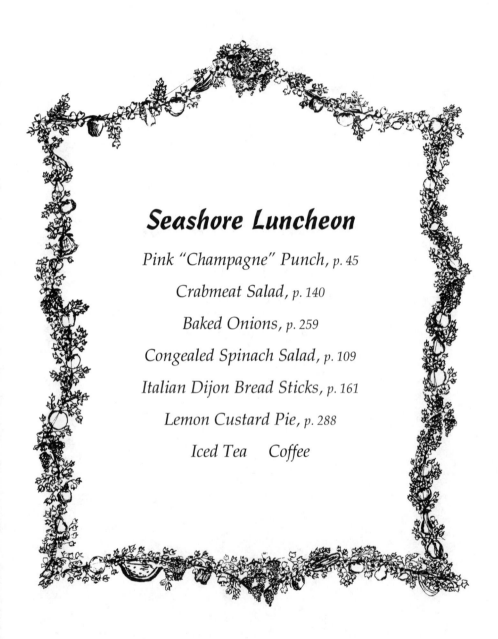

Seashore Luncheon

Pink "Champagne" Punch, p. 45

Crabmeat Salad, p. 140

Baked Onions, p. 259

Congealed Spinach Salad, p. 109

Italian Dijon Bread Sticks, p. 161

Lemon Custard Pie, p. 288

Iced Tea   Coffee

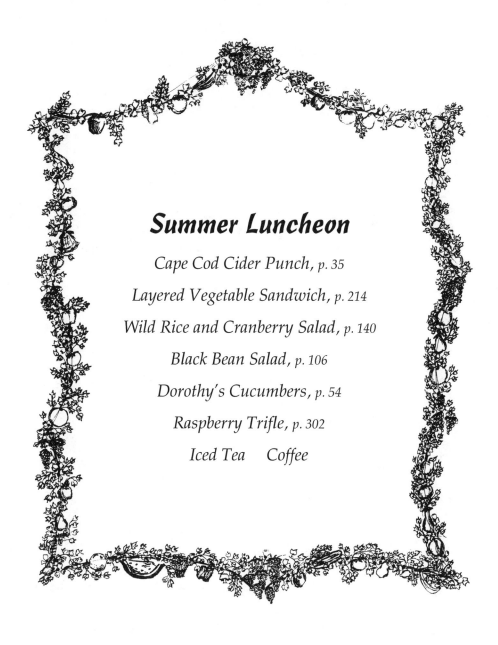

Summer Luncheon

Cape Cod Cider Punch, p. 35

Layered Vegetable Sandwich, p. 214

Wild Rice and Cranberry Salad, p. 140

Black Bean Salad, p. 106

Dorothy's Cucumbers, p. 54

Raspberry Trifle, p. 302

Iced Tea   Coffee

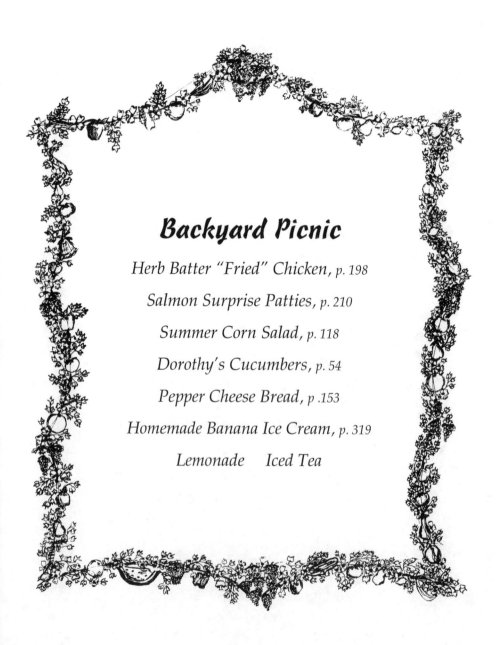

Backyard Picnic

Herb Batter "Fried" Chicken, p. 198

Salmon Surprise Patties, p. 210

Summer Corn Salad, p. 118

Dorothy's Cucumbers, p. 54

Pepper Cheese Bread, p .153

Homemade Banana Ice Cream, p. 319

Lemonade   Iced Tea

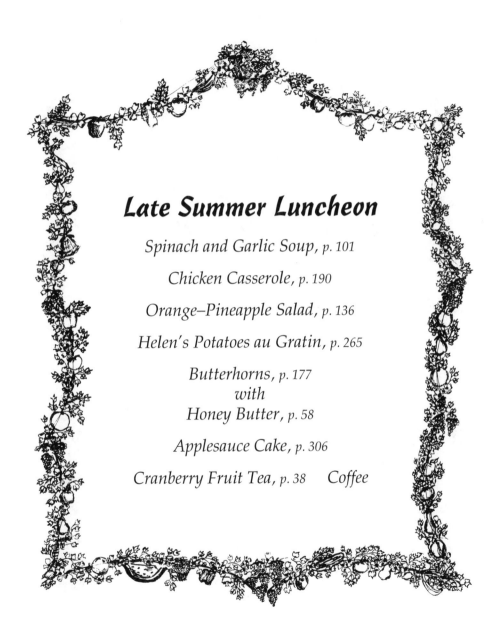

Late Summer Luncheon

Spinach and Garlic Soup, p. 101

Chicken Casserole, p. 190

Orange–Pineapple Salad, p. 136

Helen's Potatoes au Gratin, p. 265

Butterhorns, p. 177
with
Honey Butter, p. 58

Applesauce Cake, p. 306

Cranberry Fruit Tea, p. 38   *Coffee*

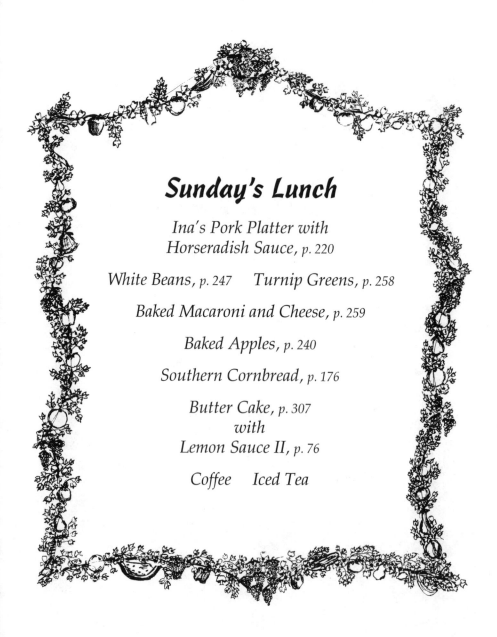

Sunday's Lunch

*Ina's Pork Platter with
Horseradish Sauce,* p. 220

White Beans, p. 247   *Turnip Greens,* p. 258

Baked Macaroni and Cheese, p. 259

Baked Apples, p. 240

Southern Cornbread, p. 176

Butter Cake, p. 307
with
Lemon Sauce II, p. 76

Coffee   Iced Tea

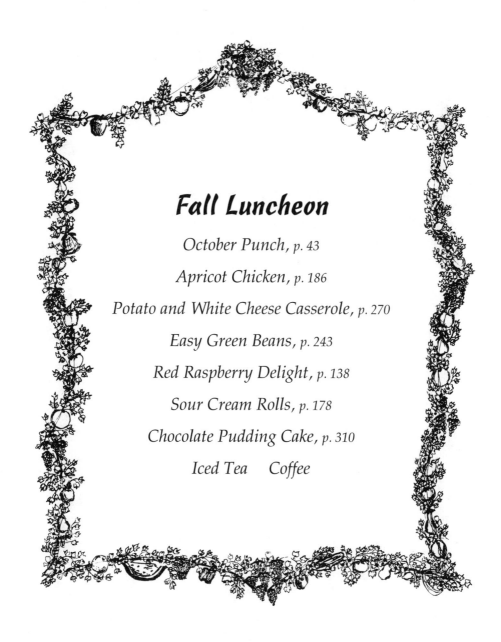

Fall Luncheon

October Punch, p. 43

Apricot Chicken, p. 186

Potato and White Cheese Casserole, p. 270

Easy Green Beans, p. 243

Red Raspberry Delight, p. 138

Sour Cream Rolls, p. 178

Chocolate Pudding Cake, p. 310

Iced Tea   Coffee

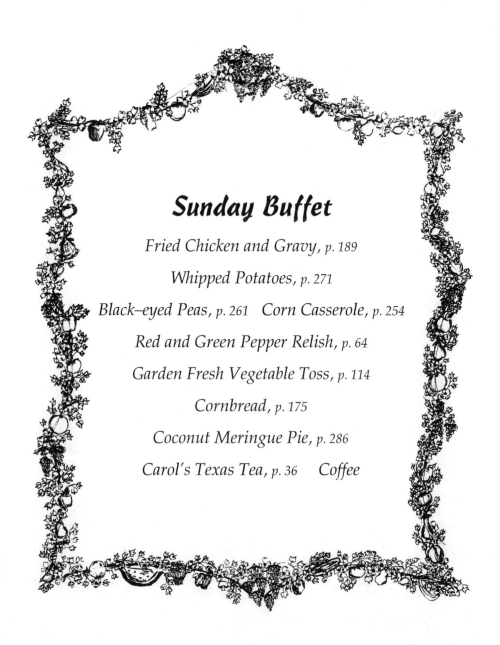

Sunday Buffet

Fried Chicken and Gravy, p. 189

Whipped Potatoes, p. 271

Black–eyed Peas, p. 261   Corn Casserole, p. 254

Red and Green Pepper Relish, p. 64

Garden Fresh Vegetable Toss, p. 114

Cornbread, p. 175

Coconut Meringue Pie, p. 286

Carol's Texas Tea, p. 36   Coffee

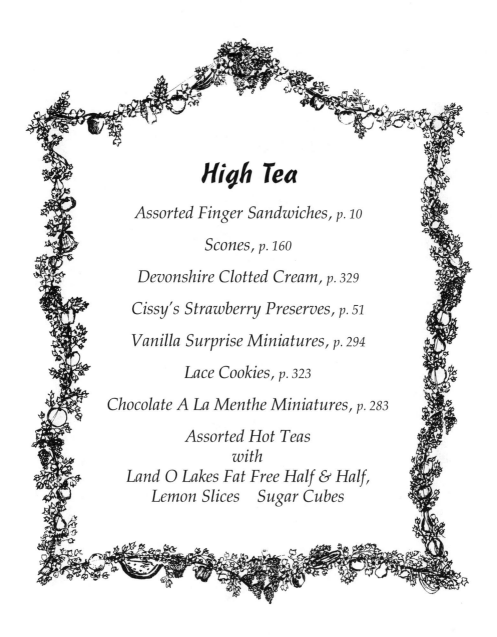

High Tea

Assorted Finger Sandwiches, p. 10

Scones, p. 160

Devonshire Clotted Cream, p. 329

Cissy's Strawberry Preserves, p. 51

Vanilla Surprise Miniatures, p. 294

Lace Cookies, p. 323

Chocolate A La Menthe Miniatures, p. 283

Assorted Hot Teas
with
Land O Lakes Fat Free Half & Half,
Lemon Slices   Sugar Cubes

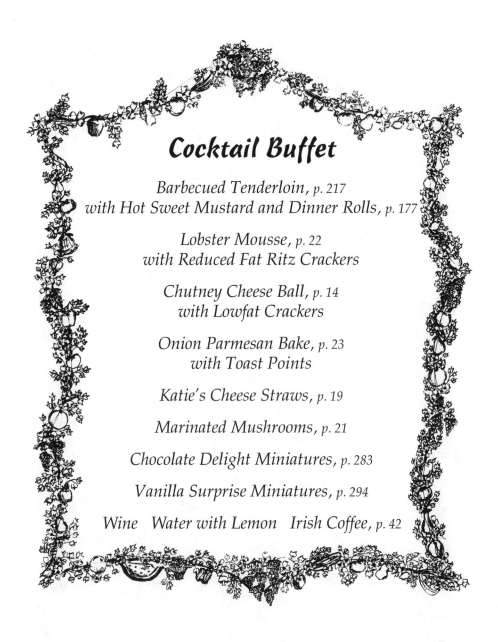

Cocktail Buffet

Barbecued Tenderloin, p. 217
with Hot Sweet Mustard and Dinner Rolls, p. 177

Lobster Mousse, p. 22
with Reduced Fat Ritz Crackers

Chutney Cheese Ball, p. 14
with Lowfat Crackers

Onion Parmesan Bake, p. 23
with Toast Points

Katie's Cheese Straws, p. 19

Marinated Mushrooms, p. 21

Chocolate Delight Miniatures, p. 283

Vanilla Surprise Miniatures, p. 294

Wine   Water with Lemon   Irish Coffee, p. 42

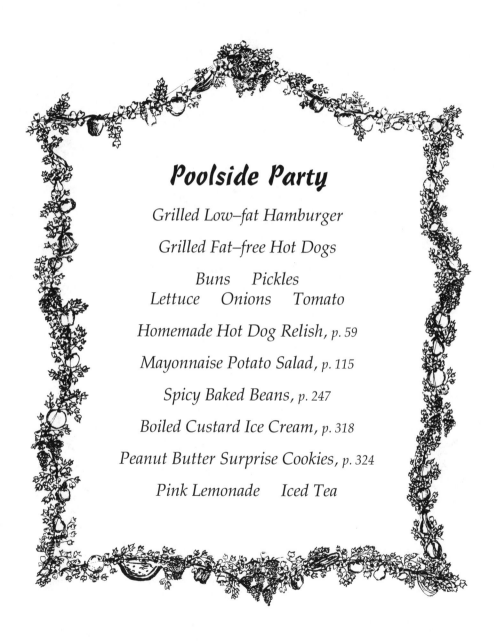

Poolside Party

Grilled Low–fat Hamburger

Grilled Fat–free Hot Dogs

Buns   Pickles
Lettuce   Onions   Tomato

Homemade Hot Dog Relish, p. 59

Mayonnaise Potato Salad, p. 115

Spicy Baked Beans, p. 247

Boiled Custard Ice Cream, p. 318

Peanut Butter Surprise Cookies, p. 324

Pink Lemonade   Iced Tea

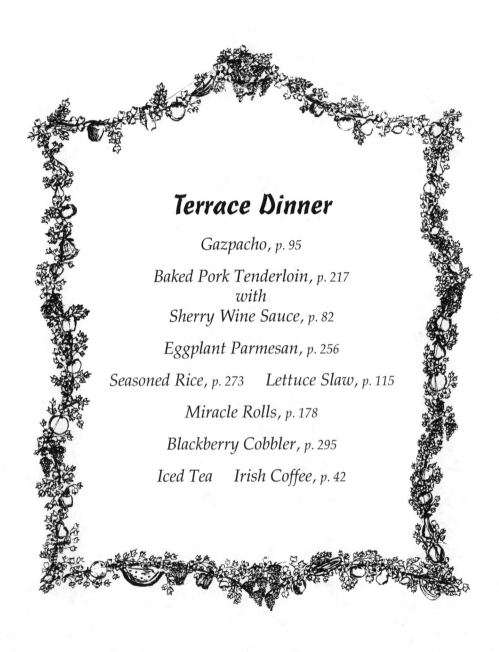

Terrace Dinner

Gazpacho, p. 95

Baked Pork Tenderloin, p. 217
with
Sherry Wine Sauce, p. 82

Eggplant Parmesan, p. 256

Seasoned Rice, p. 273   Lettuce Slaw, p. 115

Miracle Rolls, p. 178

Blackberry Cobbler, p. 295

Iced Tea   Irish Coffee, p. 42

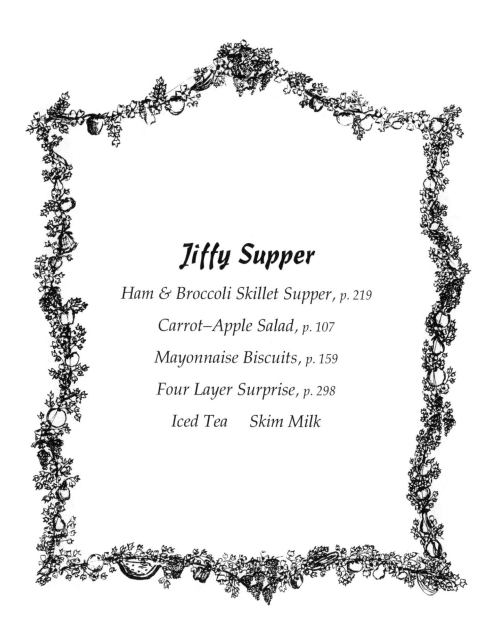

Jiffy Supper

Ham & Broccoli Skillet Supper, p. 219

Carrot–Apple Salad, p. 107

Mayonnaise Biscuits, p. 159

Four Layer Surprise, p. 298

Iced Tea   Skim Milk

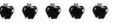
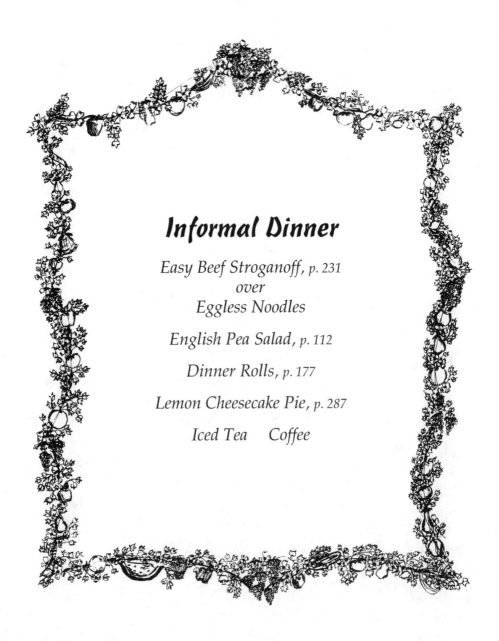

Informal Dinner

Easy Beef Stroganoff, p. 231
over
Eggless Noodles

English Pea Salad, p. 112

Dinner Rolls, p. 177

Lemon Cheesecake Pie, p. 287

Iced Tea   Coffee

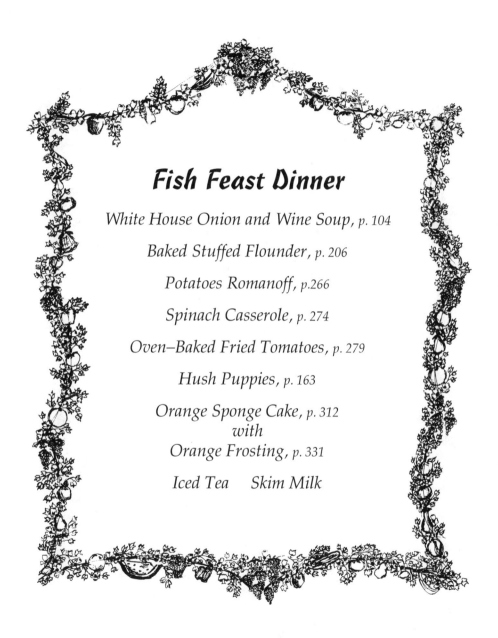

Fish Feast Dinner

White House Onion and Wine Soup, p. 104

Baked Stuffed Flounder, p. 206

Potatoes Romanoff, p.266

Spinach Casserole, p. 274

Oven–Baked Fried Tomatoes, p. 279

Hush Puppies, p. 163

Orange Sponge Cake, p. 312
with
Orange Frosting, p. 331

Iced Tea   Skim Milk

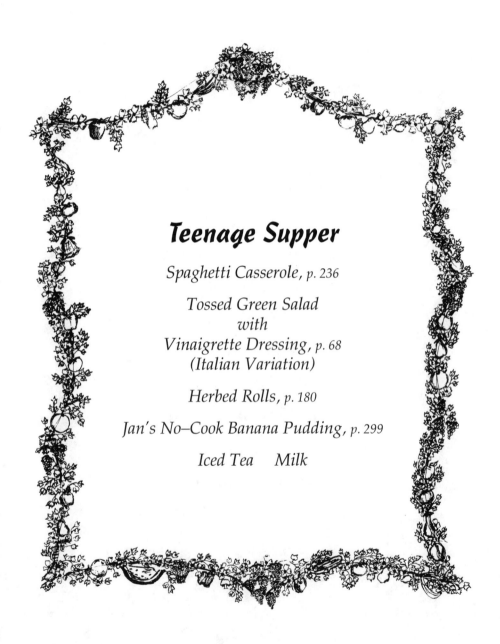

Teenage Supper

Spaghetti Casserole, p. 236

Tossed Green Salad
with
Vinaigrette Dressing, p. 68
(Italian Variation)

Herbed Rolls, p. 180

Jan's No–Cook Banana Pudding, p. 299

Iced Tea   Milk

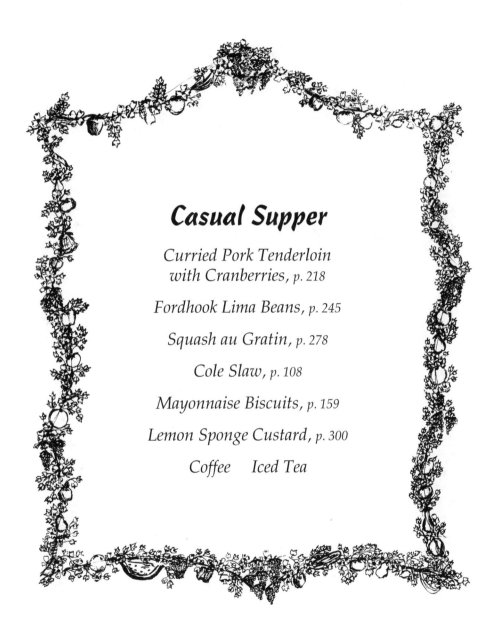

Casual Supper

*Curried Pork Tenderloin
with Cranberries,* p. 218

Fordhook Lima Beans, p. 245

Squash au Gratin, p. 278

Cole Slaw, p. 108

Mayonnaise Biscuits, p. 159

Lemon Sponge Custard, p. 300

Coffee   Iced Tea

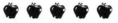

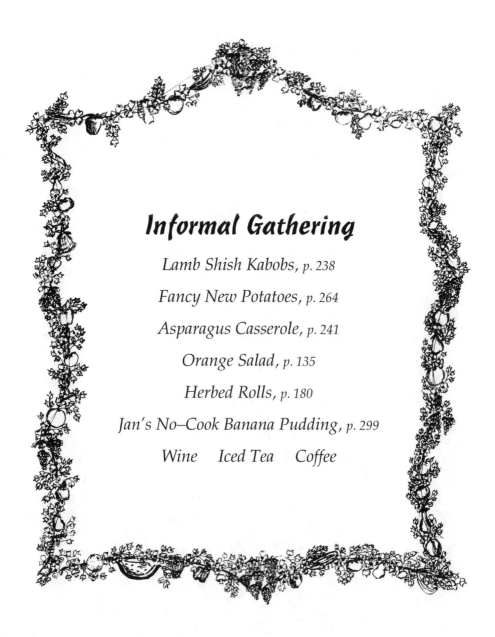

Informal Gathering

Lamb Shish Kabobs, p. 238

Fancy New Potatoes, p. 264

Asparagus Casserole, p. 241

Orange Salad, p. 135

Herbed Rolls, p. 180

Jan's No–Cook Banana Pudding, p. 299

Wine   Iced Tea   Coffee

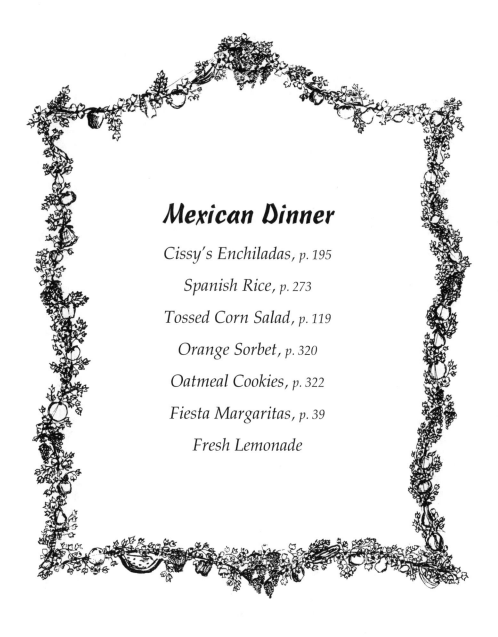

Mexican Dinner

Cissy's Enchiladas, p. 195

Spanish Rice, p. 273

Tossed Corn Salad, p. 119

Orange Sorbet, p. 320

Oatmeal Cookies, p. 322

Fiesta Margaritas, p. 39

Fresh Lemonade

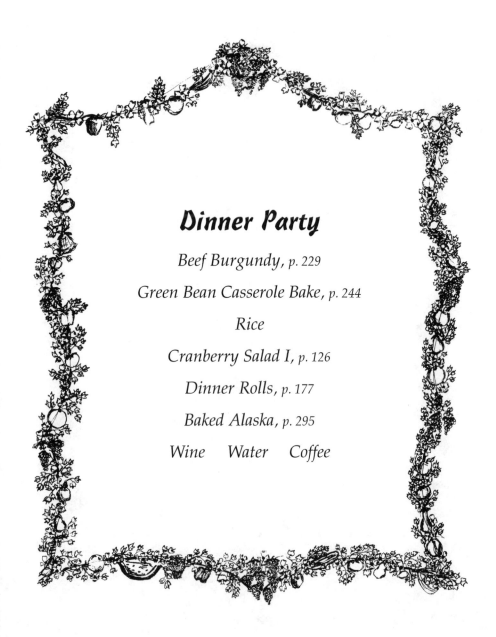

Dinner Party

Beef Burgundy, p. 229

Green Bean Casserole Bake, p. 244

Rice

Cranberry Salad I, p. 126

Dinner Rolls, p. 177

Baked Alaska, p. 295

Wine   Water   Coffee

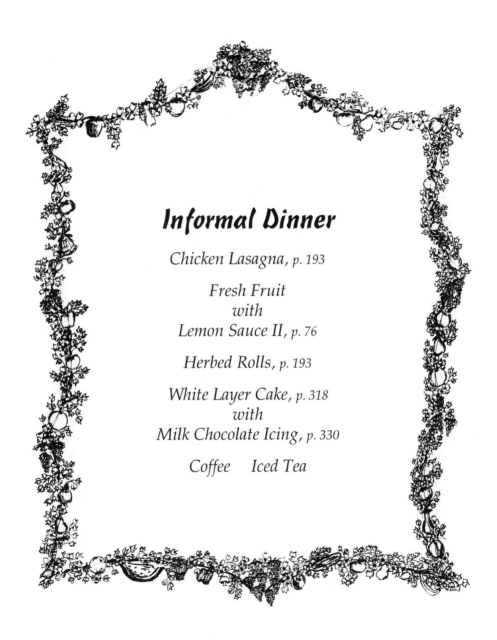

Informal Dinner

Chicken Lasagna, p. 193

Fresh Fruit
with
Lemon Sauce II, p. 76

Herbed Rolls, p. 193

White Layer Cake, p. 318
with
Milk Chocolate Icing, p. 330

Coffee   Iced Tea

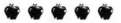
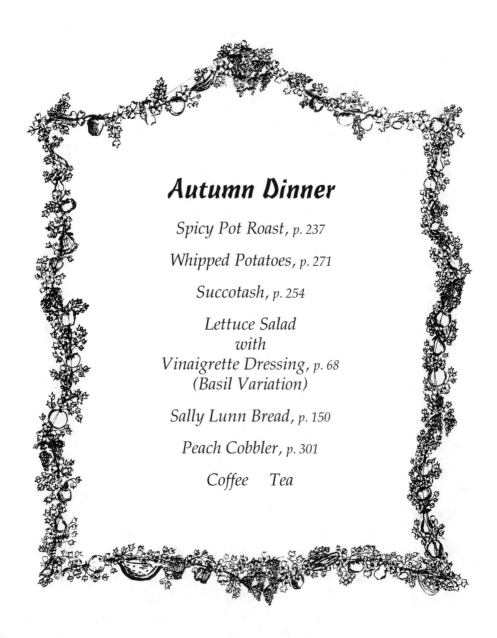

Autumn Dinner

Spicy Pot Roast, p. 237

Whipped Potatoes, p. 271

Succotash, p. 254

*Lettuce Salad
with
Vinaigrette Dressing*, p. 68
(Basil Variation)

Sally Lunn Bread, p. 150

Peach Cobbler, p. 301

Coffee   Tea

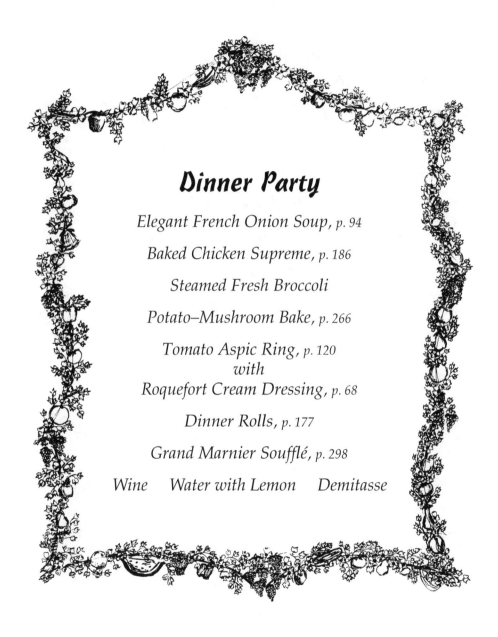

Dinner Party

Elegant French Onion Soup, p. 94

Baked Chicken Supreme, p. 186

Steamed Fresh Broccoli

Potato–Mushroom Bake, p. 266

Tomato Aspic Ring, p. 120
with
Roquefort Cream Dressing, p. 68

Dinner Rolls, p. 177

Grand Marnier Soufflé, p. 298

Wine   Water with Lemon   Demitasse

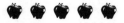
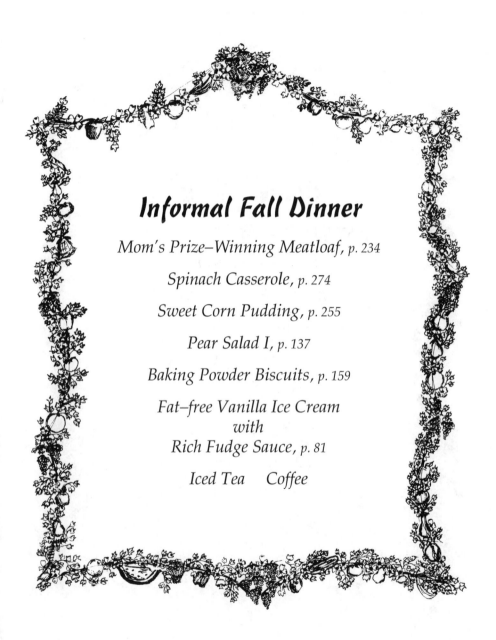

Informal Fall Dinner

Mom's Prize–Winning Meatloaf, p. 234

Spinach Casserole, p. 274

Sweet Corn Pudding, p. 255

Pear Salad I, p. 137

Baking Powder Biscuits, p. 159

Fat–free Vanilla Ice Cream
with
Rich Fudge Sauce, p. 81

Iced Tea   Coffee

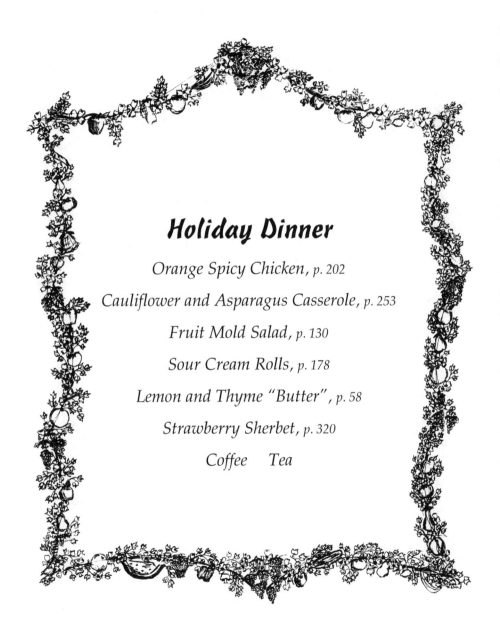

Holiday Dinner

Orange Spicy Chicken, p. 202

Cauliflower and Asparagus Casserole, p. 253

Fruit Mold Salad, p. 130

Sour Cream Rolls, p. 178

Lemon and Thyme "Butter", p. 58

Strawberry Sherbet, p. 320

Coffee   Tea

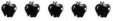
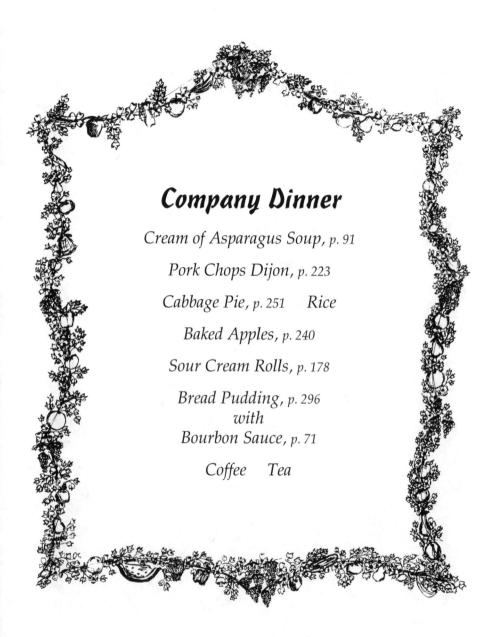

Company Dinner

Cream of Asparagus Soup, p. 91

Pork Chops Dijon, p. 223

Cabbage Pie, p. 251   Rice

Baked Apples, p. 240

Sour Cream Rolls, p. 178

Bread Pudding, p. 296
with
Bourbon Sauce, p. 71

Coffee   Tea

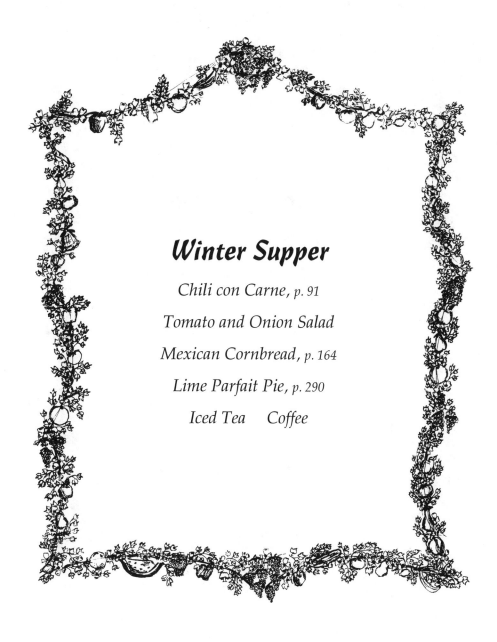

Winter Supper

Chili con Carne, p. 91

Tomato and Onion Salad

Mexican Cornbread, p. 164

Lime Parfait Pie, p. 290

Iced Tea   Coffee

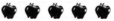

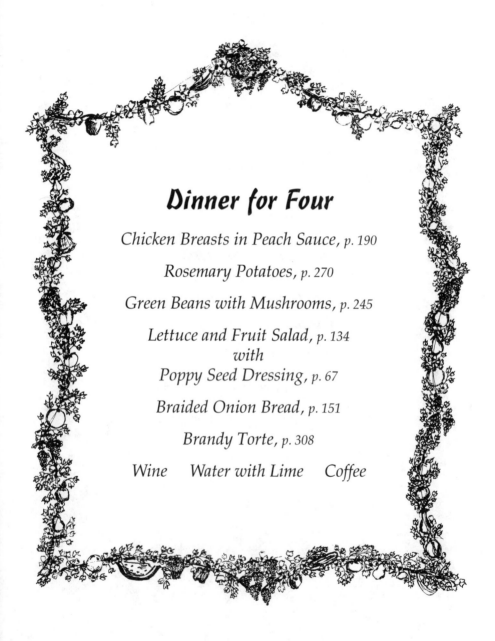

Dinner for Four

Chicken Breasts in Peach Sauce, p. 190

Rosemary Potatoes, p. 270

Green Beans with Mushrooms, p. 245

Lettuce and Fruit Salad, p. 134
with
Poppy Seed Dressing, p. 67

Braided Onion Bread, p. 151

Brandy Torte, p. 308

Wine   Water with Lime   Coffee

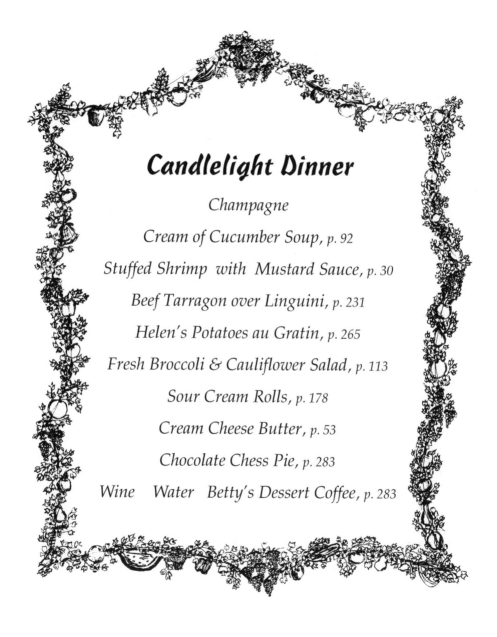

Candlelight Dinner

Champagne

Cream of Cucumber Soup, p. 92

Stuffed Shrimp with Mustard Sauce, p. 30

Beef Tarragon over Linguini, p. 231

Helen's Potatoes au Gratin, p. 265

Fresh Broccoli & Cauliflower Salad, p. 113

Sour Cream Rolls, p. 178

Cream Cheese Butter, p. 53

Chocolate Chess Pie, p. 283

Wine   Water   Betty's Dessert Coffee, p. 283

Notes

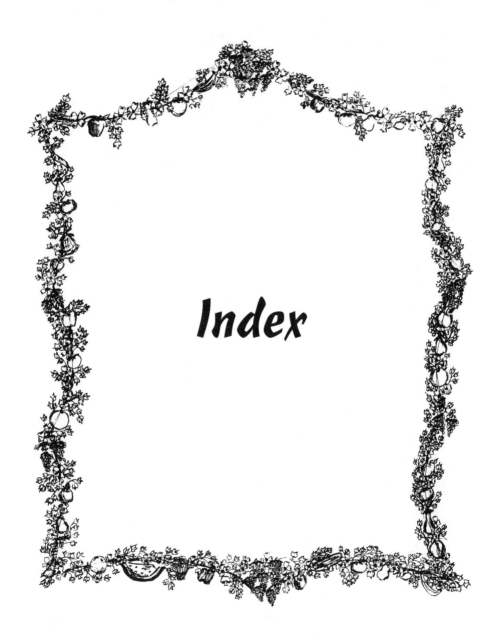

Index

C

CONDIMENTS

Index 🍎 🍎 🍎 🍎 🍎

D

DESSERTS

M

MAIN DISHES

Index 🍎 🍎 🍎 🍎 🍎

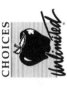

CHOICES
Unlimited®

YES! Tell me more about

Please send me:

_____ Information about Choices Unlimited Workshops.

_____ Information on arranging for a Choices Unlimited Lecture for my organization.

_____ Copy(s) of the *Fite For Your Life* Cookbook at $16.95 plus $4.00 tax, shipping and handling, each.

_____ Copy(s) of the *Fite For Your Life II* Cookbook at $19.95 plus $4.50 tax, shipping and handling, each.

_____ Copy(s) of the *Fite For Your Life* Video Set $29.95 plus $6.50 tax, shipping and handling, per set.

Name _____

Address _____

_____

Phone _____

Make all checks payable to Choices Unlimited, Inc.

For Credit Card orders:

☐ MasterCard   ☐ Visa

Card No. _____

Expiration Date _____

Signature _____

Mail to: Choices Unlimited, Inc.
89 Stonehaven Drive
Jackson, TN 38305
Phone (901) 664-6707

Reorder Additional Copies